AF676206

Medical Discourse in Professional, Academic and Popular Settings

MIX
Paper from
responsible sources
FSC® C013604

LANGUAGE AT WORK

Series Editors**: Jo Angouri**, *University of Warwick, UK* and **Rebecca Piekkari**, *Aalto University Business School, Finland*

Language at Work is a new series designed to bring together scholars interested in workplace research. The modern workplace has changed significantly in recent years. The international nature of business activities and the increasing rate of mobility around the world create a new challenging environment for individuals and organisations alike. The advancements in technology have reshaped the ways employees collaborate at the interface of linguistic, national and professional borders. The complex linguistic landscape also results in new challenges for health care systems and legal settings. This and other phenomena around the world of work have attracted significant interest; it is still common however for relevant research to remain within clear disciplinary and methodological boundaries.

The series aims to create space for exchange of ideas and dialogue and seeks to explore issues related to power, leadership, politics, teamwork, culture, ideology, identity, decision making and motivation across a diverse range of contexts, including corporate, health care and institutional settings. *Language at Work* welcomes mixed methods research and it will be of interest to researchers in linguistics, international management, organisation studies, sociology, medical sociology and decision sciences.

Full details of all the books in this series and of all our other publications can be found on http://www.multilingual-matters.com, or by writing to Multilingual Matters, St Nicholas House, 31-34 High Street, Bristol BS1 2AW, UK

LANGUAGE AT WORK: 1

Medical Discourse in Professional, Academic and Popular Settings

Edited by

Pilar Ordóñez-López
Nuria Edo-Marzá

MULTILINGUAL MATTERS
Bristol • Buffalo • Toronto

Library of Congress Cataloging in Publication Data
A catalog record for this book is available from the Library of Congress.
Names: Ordóñez López, Pilar, editor. | Edo-Marzá, Nuria, editor.
Title: Medical discourse in professional, academic and popular settings / edited by Pilar Ordóñez López and Nuria Edo- Marzá.
Description: Bristol; Buffalo: Multilingual Matters [2016] | Series: Language At Work: 1 | Includes bibliographical references and index.
Identifiers: LCCN 2016022310| ISBN 9781783096251 (hbk : alk. paper) | ISBN 9781783096275 (epub) | ISBN 9781783096282 (kindle)
Subjects: LCSH: Discourse analysis. | Communication in medicine. | Medicine--Language. | Language in the workplace--Social aspects. | Sociolinguistics.
Classification: LCC P302 .M3924 2016 | DDC 610.1/41--dc23 LC record available at https://lccn.loc.gov/2016022310

British Library Cataloguing in Publication Data
A catalogue entry for this book is available from the British Library.

ISBN-13: 978-1-78309-625-1 (hbk)

Multilingual Matters
UK: St Nicholas House, 31-34 High Street, Bristol BS1 2AW, UK.
USA: UTP, 2250 Military Road, Tonawanda, NY 14150, USA.
Canada: UTP, 5201 Dufferin Street, North York, Ontario M3H 5T8, Canada.

Website: www.multilingual-matters.com
Twitter: Multi_Ling_Mat
Facebook: https://www.facebook.com/multilingualmatters
Blog: www.channelviewpublications.wordpress.com

Copyright © 2016 Pilar Ordóñez-López, Nuria Edo-Marzá and the authors of individual chapters.

All rights reserved. No part of this work may be reproduced in any form or by any means without permission in writing from the publisher.

The policy of Multilingual Matters/Channel View Publications is to use papers that are natural, renewable and recyclable products, made from wood grown in sustainable forests. In the manufacturing process of our books, and to further support our policy, preference is given to printers that have FSC and PEFC Chain of Custody certification. The FSC and/or PEFC logos will appear on those books where full certification has been granted to the printer concerned.

Typeset by Deanta Global Publishing Services Limited.
Printed and bound by CPI Group (UK) Ltd, Croydon, CR0 4YY

Contents

Contributors

Begoña Bellés Fortuño holds a PhD in English Philology from Jaume I University in Castellón, Spain, where she is Senior Lecturer in the Department of English Studies and member of the IULMA (Instituto Interuniversitario de Lenguas ModernasAplicadas). In 2006/2007, she was a Morley Scholar for the ELI (English Language Institute) at the University of Michigan (Ann Arbor, MI), where she worked together with the MICASE team. Her research interests are focused on discourse analysis, and more specifically, written and spoken academic discourse, as well as on contrastive analysis and corpus linguistics.

Martí Domínguez is Professor of Journalism in the Department of Theory of Languages at the University of Valencia, Spain. He holds a PhD in Biology and has a background as researcher in media and science communication. He leads The Two Cultures Observatory, a multidisciplinary research group of the University of Valencia that focuses on the relationships between scientists and the media. He has published widely in the areas of visual communication, metaphors and knowledge exchange between scientists and the public.

Nuria Edo-Marzá is Assistant Professor in the Department of English Studies at Jaume I University in Castellón, Spain, as well as a member of the IULMA (Instituto Interuniversitario de Lenguas Modernas Aplicadas). Her main research areas are specialised languages, mainly those of health, science and technology, and tourism; specialised lexicography; corpus linguistics and terminology. She is the author of *The Specialised Lexicographical Approach: A Step Further in Dictionary-Making* (2009) and has published in international journals and volumes. As regards medical language, she is the author of *Spoken English for the Medical Professional* (2012), *English for Patient Administration and Non-Clinical Hospital Staff* (2011) and *English for Pharmacists* (2011), and has co-authored a chapter entitled 'The peer reviewing process in medical research: Positive and negative effects on scientific advancement', included in the international volume *The Language of Health Care* (2008).

Isabel García-Izquierdo is Professor of Linguistics Applied to Translation and of Spanish for Translators in the Department of Translation and Communication at Jaume I University in Castellón, Spain. Since 2000, she has been the director of the research group GENTT (Textual Genres for Translation), which focuses on multilingual analysis of textual genres in the framework of specialised communication applied to translation. She is a member of the IULMA (Instituto Interuniversitario de Lenguas Modernas Aplicadas). Isabel García-Izquierdo has published several books as well as articles in national and international journals such as *Sendebar, Hermeneus, Trans, Iberica, Meta, ITT, Target, Linguistica Antverpiensia*. She is the author of *Análisis textual aplicado a la Traducción* (2000), *Divulgación médica y traducción. El género Información para pacientes* (2010) and *Competencia textual para la traducción* (2011); she is also the editor of *El género textual y la traducción* (2005) and co-editor of *Iberian Studies on Translation and Interpreting. New Trends in Translation Studies*, Vol. 11 (2012).

Maurizio Gotti is Professor of English Language and Translation, Head of the Department of Foreign Languages, Literatures and Cultures, and Director of the Research Centre on Specialized Languages (CERLIS) at the University of Bergamo. His main research areas are the features and origins of specialised discourse (*Robert Boyle and the Language of Science*, 1996; *Specialized Discourse: Linguistic Features and Changing Conventions*, 2003; *Investigating Specialized Discourse*, 2011). He is also interested in English syntax, English lexicology and lexicography, and in the history of the English language. He is a member of the editorial board of national and international journals, and edits the *Linguistic Insights* series for Peter Lang.

Vicent Montalt Resurrecció is Senior Lecturer and teaches medical, scientific and technical translation at Jaume I University in Castellón, Spain. He is the director of the Master in Medical Translation and of the research group *TradMed* that works on medical translation, as well as being a member of the research group GENTT (Textual Genres for Translation) and of the IULMA (Instituto Interuniversitario de Lenguas Modernas Aplicadas). He is the author of *Manual de traducció cientificotècnica* (2005) and co-author of *Medical Translation Step by Step. Learning by Drafting* (2007).

Ignasi Navarro i Ferrando holds a PhD in English linguistics. After graduating from the University of Valencia in Hispanic Studies as well as English Studies, he taught at the University of Mainz in 1989–1990, and since 1991 at Jaume I University, where he is currently Senior Lecturer in the Department of English Studies. He is a member of the IULMA (Instituto Interuniversitario de Lenguas Modernas Aplicadas). His co-edited books include *Los Estilos de Aprendizaje de Lenguas: Representaciones Culturales e Interacciones de Enseñanza-Aprendizaje* (1997), *Cognitive and Discourse*

Approaches to Metaphor and Metonymy (2005) and *Sistemas lingüísticos y perspectiva cognitiva* (2010). He is co-author of *Culturas Cara a Cara. Relatos y Actividades para la Comunicación Intercultural* (2006).

Pilar Ordóñez-López is Lecturer in Translation Studies at Jaume I University in Castellón (Spain), where she teaches Translation Theory and Legal Translation. She is a member of the IULMA (Instituto Interuniversitario de Lenguas Modernas Aplicadas). Her research interests include the history of translation, translation theory, corpus-based translation studies and legal translation, and she has published widely in these areas. Among her most relevant publications, a monograph on Ortega y Gasset's views on translation (2009), a study of translation anthologies in Spain and Portugal (2012, with Sabio Pinilla) and a reader on Iberian translation historiography (2015, with Sabio Pinilla) can be cited. She is also an official sworn translator, appointed by the Spanish Ministry of Foreign Affairs.

Morten Pilegaard is Associate Professor of Language for Special Purposes in the Department of Business Communication, Faculty of Business and Social Sciences, Aarhus University, Denmark, as well as Director of Knowledge Communication Lab, Aarhus University, and he is also Director and Partner of TermShare A/S. His main research areas are English for Academic Purposes in general and the language of medicine and life sciences in particular (Informed consent: Towards improved lay-friendliness of patient information sheets, *Communication and Medicine* 2014; Readability of patient information can be improved, *Danish Medical Bulletin* 2011), as well as academic entrepreneurship and knowledge sharing (An auto-ethnographic perspective on academic entrepreneurship: Implications for research in the social sciences and humanities, *Academy of Management Perspectives* 2010). He has served as terminology advisor to the Danish National Board of Health, as a professor with special responsibilities for the Danish Business Research Academy and is currently a consultant on medical language for the Danish Medical Association, among others. He has been working in the domain of medical language for the past 30 years.

Vicent Salvador is Professor in the Department of Philology and European Cultures at Jaume I University in Castellón (Spain) and a member of the IULMA (Instituto Interuniversitario de Lenguas Modernas Aplicadas). His research interests include discourse analysis and literary theory. Some of his most relevant publications are 'Un nuevo modelo de discurso biográfico: los casos clínicos literaturizados de Oliver Sacks' (2015), in Balaguer *et al.*, *Aproximació a l'altre: Biografies, semblances i retrats* (Amsterdam: J. Benjamins) and 'Autorrelato e identidades profesionales: sobre autobiografías de científicos y médicos'(2015), *Annali de Ca' Foscari. Serie Occidentale*, 49.

He is also co-director of the journal *Cultura, Lenguaje y Representación/ Culture, Language and Representation.*

Lucía Sapiña holds a bachelor degree in communication studies and a master in history of science and scientific communication. She is a PhD candidate at the López Piñero Institute for the History of Medicine and Science at the University of Valencia, Spain. She also works as a researcher in The Two Cultures Observatory. Her research interests include cancer in the media, as well as the transmission of scientific and medical knowledge to a wider audience.

Antonio-José Silvestre-López is Assistant Professor in the Department of English Studies at Jaume I University in Castellón, Spain, from which he also received his PhD with European Honours in Applied Linguistics. He is a member of the IULMA (Instituto Interuniversitario de Lenguas Modernas Aplicadas). His main research interests are the study of particle semantics from a cognitive perspective and the use of corpora in EFL contexts. Recently, he has also developed an interest in the identification of sets of Idealised Cognitive Models (ICMs) for the conceptualisation of subjective (first-person) experiences derived from mindfulness meditation practices and their (third-person) communication in instructional settings via the analysis of the oral production of novice and experienced practitioners.

1 Medical Discourse: Building Bridges between Medicine and Society

Pilar Ordóñez-López
Nuria Edo-Marzá

Medical discourse not only allows medical professionals to communicate among each other, but it is also the link between the medical profession and the public, including patients. As pointed out by scholars such as Gotti and Salager-Meyer (2006: 10), medicine has always occupied a prominent place in all cultures and times, for the simple reason that it affects the health and lives of all human beings. Furthermore, as shown by the growing number of medical journals as well as non-medical journals devoted to the study of medical discourse, medical communication has become a cornerstone of our society. Access to specialised discourse is no longer restricted to the privileged few (Pilegaard, 2007) and, as Weingart (2002: 704) observes, by entering the public arena, knowledge, in this case medical knowledge, is subjected to the judgement and evaluation of society. The need to communicate, to take into consideration the other (the patient, the medical student, the general public, etc.), the need to be aware of the ethical implications involved and to become conscious of the factors which are decisive in order for communication to be successful – all of these are key aspects for the achievement of successful communication, for establishing a fruitful and dynamic dialogue between science, i.e. medicine, and society. On the other hand, these issues have no doubt contributed to the increasing interest in the study of medical discourse in a wide variety of settings and from a wide range of perspectives.

Another key issue in today's medical discourse, closely related to the aspects mentioned above, is popularisation, aimed at making specialised, medical knowledge accessible to the layman. According to Gotti (2014: 19), popularisation has greatly influenced the discourse of medicine, enhancing both new textual realisations (e.g. genres such as popular science articles) and new formats for the dissemination and sharing of knowledge (not only limited to specialised journals and forums, but also the media and other formats available and easily accessible to the general public).

Gotti's (2014) work reveals the complexity of this phenomenon, which involves reformulation and recontextualisation, in order to guarantee that information is successfully transferred. These processes, in turn, favour certain linguistic, textual and cognitive mechanisms, such as the use of metaphors (Gotti, 2014: 28), aiming to facilitate the general public's understanding of the specialised (medical) content by constructing an informative and explanatory discourse. The popularisation of medical discourse, at the same time, implies paying attention to non-experts, e.g. the patient, leading to the analysis of the ethical issues arising from the access to and (mis)understanding of medical content by the public.

The shift of emphasis towards patient-centred healthcare has triggered interest in communication issues, which, as pointed out by Sarangi (2012: 13), has resulted in the incorporation of the teaching of communication skills within the medical training context. This new perspective has also brought about a shift in communication, as explained by Montalt and Shuttleworth (2012), from a monologic paradigm (in which the only voice worth listening to was the doctor's) to a dialogic one. Furthermore, the acknowledgement of the need to promote fruitful and dynamic interaction (doctor–patient) in order to successfully communicate has caused scholars to consider oral discourse a nuclear aspect, and it is the object of a significant amount of research in a wide range of contexts (e.g. Bowles, 2006; Candlin, 2006; Cordella, 2004; García-Izquierdo & Montalt, 2013).

Another trend that has shaped the discourse of medicine in recent years is the incorporation of complementary and alternative medicine (often referred to as CAM), which has become increasingly popular in Western societies in recent decades (cf., e.g. Gale & McHale, 2015; Salager-Meyer *et al.*, 2006; Sharma, 2000). This is also an indication of the shifting focus in the medical context and has been reflected in the consideration of the notion of health from a more integrative, holistic and patient-oriented perspective. In sum, this is another example of how the present-day discourse of medicine is encouraging dialogue between diverse perspectives and is becoming an increasingly integrative area of knowledge, aware of the importance of meeting the needs of society.

The discourse of medicine is thus interactive and social, and as such it is critical for both the medical professional and the linguist to know how it is articulated and shaped to achieve successful communication, according to the different aims and settings involved. The study of medical discourse has gradually incorporated new perspectives resulting from the integration of input from other related fields, such as applied linguistics, sociology, corpus linguistics and cognitive linguistics. This has been possible thanks to the incorporation of some key theoretical perspectives, such as the study of genres and the use of corpora, as well as the focus on realia, i.e. the study of real cases, real contexts and real instances of medical communication, be it among medical professionals, doctors and patients, the media, etc.

This volume provides a multidisciplinary study of medical discourse based on corpus-driven investigations, carried out within different theoretical frameworks (e.g. sociology, corpus linguistics), applied both to individual case studies and more general linguistic, textual and discourse-specific analyses of medical communication. The contributions included in this book deal with key aspects of medical discourse, such as the use of metaphor referring to cancer, the importance of ethics in medical documents addressed to patients and the linguistic challenges involved, as well as the discourse analysis of some fundamental medical genres. Though diverse and wide-ranging, the contributions have in common that they adopt a comprehensive and up-to-date perspective, from which the rhetoric of medicine is examined in key settings (the media, academic and educational contexts, instances of real doctor–patient interaction, etc.) providing interesting new insights into the study of medical discourse.

Gotti presents a corpus-based study of variation in medical discourse for academic purposes, focusing on the relation between socioculturally oriented identity factors and textual variation. He reviews some current research projects devoted to the examination of identity-forming features linked to 'local' or disciplinary cultures through the analysis of specialised discourse in English in various academic domains by native and non-native speakers. He also discusses the results obtained in the CERLIS project, aimed at investigating to what extent the cultural allegiance of (native or non-native) anglophone discourse communities to their linguistic, professional, social or national reference groups is affected by the use of English as a lingua franca of international communication. This study shows the influence of factors such as the affiliation of writers to different professional, ideological or ethnic-geographic cultures on the realisation of medical discourse in academic settings.

The contributions by Salvador and Bellés-Fortuño deal with different medical genres, paying special attention to the training context, and they underline the importance of developing communication skills in the professionals of the future.

Salvador's chapter explores how the case study in medical and health settings (clinical case report [CCR]) is a regular section in some specialised academic periodicals, despite the controversy about its scientific nature. The author claims that the analysis of clinical cases as an actual instance of a therapeutic process is especially relevant in the study of *communities of practice*, a conceptual framework related to the sociology of professional training. According to Salvador, the prevalence of the narrative dimension in clinical cases has the potential to make the professional experience accessible and convey it to readers. The author explores the structure and content of CCRs, concluding that the CCR, as a medical narrative, contributes to the construction of the patient's identity. The inclusion of the CCR as a genre in medical journals counteracts the tendency towards a mere scientific biomedicine by providing a new perspective on more human-centred and personalised, yet scientific, health studies, capable of building bridges between science and the humanities.

Also with a focus on the educational context, Bellés-Fortuño provides a corpus-based analysis of two medical genres (scientific research articles and popular science articles), aiming to show the suitability of popular science articles for medical students. The author undertakes a contrastive study of the structure and use of evaluative language and linguistic features such as discourse markers in both genres, based on an ad hoc corpus of articles on the same topic (arthritis) extracted from the website *Science Daily* and the medical journal *The Lancet*. The results obtained allow the author to conclude that popular science articles, which tend to be simpler and shorter than scientific research articles, can be used as pedagogical tools to promote more intuitive learning and facilitate students' understanding of medical discourse, especially in their first years of education, when they tend to find the reading of research articles arduous.

Pilegaard's and Montalt & García-Izquierdo's chapters focus on textual genres addressed to patients with the aim of providing new insights into the ethicalness of informed consent documents (ICDs) and compare oral and written modes of communication, underlining the challenges posed by these genres for translators and writers of medical texts.

In his contribution, Pilegaard focuses on ethical issues involved in healthcare and claims that it is necessary to adopt a patient-centred approach and tailor communication to the patient's specific knowledge level and information needs. From an integrative perspective, Pilegaard advocates a model of analysis which builds on systemic functional linguistics (SFL) and incorporates aspects of other applied linguistics disciplines, such as genre theory, translation theory and discourse analysis, in order to cover all the dimensions that have an impact on ethicalness. The author carries out a multidimensional analysis of real ICDs, used to obtain consent for the participation in medical research in Denmark. The results obtained reveal a general lack of ethicalness: structural patterns are not always appropriate; the choice of lexical items shows a lack of consideration of the reader's knowledge level; the reader tends to be described as an object of investigation rather than an individual addressee; and the use of officialese and other expert language features creates distance between the expert and the layman (the addressee). All these aspects are detrimental to an ethical doctor–patient interaction and hinder fluent communication in the context of medical research.

Montalt and García-Izquierdo's chapter delves into oral and written modes from a holistic and comprehensive perspective and presents proposals that strengthen the links between the two modes of communication, so as to enhance doctor–patient interaction. The study departs from a translation studies perspective, the starting point being the recognition of the possible cultural and conceptual asymmetries between patients and doctors. The authors note that more progress has been made in the study and optimisation of oral than of written communication, focusing, in the final part, on the Calgary-Cambridge Guide (CCG). Arguing that some asymmetries may be better resolved through the written mode, the authors explore the convergences and divergences between the oral genre 'consultation' and contributions based on research on written communication.

Both Navarro and Domínguez & Sapiña deal with the use of metaphors for cancer in medical discourse: while Navarro provides a comparative analysis of the use of metaphor in three medical genres, Domínguez and Sapiña analyse the use of sports metaphors for this disease in the Spanish press.

Based on corpus containing texts belonging to three different genres that frequently deal with cancer issues, namely research papers, scientific news notices and press articles, Navarro's chapter tries to unravel certain aspects of the use of metaphors in medical discourse. With this aim, the author introduces different perspectives on the notion of metaphor, followed by a characterisation of types within Conceptual Metaphor Theory (CMT) in terms of correspondences between domains. The chapter proceeds by exploring and discussing cognitive functions of metaphor, such as categorisation and conceptualisation, as well as discourse communicative functions, such as deliberate and novel usage. Furthermore, the cognitive and communicative functions of conventional metaphors in a set of genres of medical discourse are illustrated and discussed. The author presents a characterisation of the three genres analysed in terms of metaphor usage and function, so as to determine the role of metaphorical models in scientific communication. The study suggests that metaphorical usage may be more or less conscious and deliberate depending on genre and it analyses the functions metaphors fulfil in each particular one.

Domínguez and Sapiña explore the use of metaphors in medical discourse on cancer in the Spanish press and how they contribute to the creation of a collective image of the illness. The authors examine the use of cancer metaphors in a corpus consisting of news items about three events related to celebrities of Futbol Club Barcelona, published in six of the most widely read general newspapers and four of the most popular sports journals, in order to determine which type of metaphor is most frequent. Domínguez and Sapiña claim that war metaphors convey a set of negative images, such as the inevitable need to fight a battle or the annihilation of the defeated, which to some extent underline the possibility of defeat and put pressure on the cancer patient. Nevertheless, as shown in this contribution, war metaphors prevail in the discourse about cancer in the press, even in the sports context, where we might expect sports metaphors to be more common. The authors advocate the replacement of war metaphors by sports metaphors, which create a more encouraging imagery for those affected by the disease.

Finally, Silvestre-López's contribution also underlines the relevance of metaphor in the discourse of mindfulness through the analysis of the linguistic production of a target group in order to identify more effective mindfulness teaching procedures. Mindfulness is a health-related area that has experienced a great expansion in recent times, especially in the fields of psychology, psychiatry and neuroscience. Mindfulness focuses on processes of attention and the perception of sensations, emotions and thoughts. Mindfulness meditation has become a fully accepted procedure in experimental and clinical psychology to treat a range of health conditions like stress, anxiety and depression. However, as the author points out, the linguistic dimension of mindfulness still requires an in-depth investigation; a first step in that direction is taken in this chapter with the study of metaphor as a necessary tool to apprehend, mentally represent and 'handle' the above-mentioned sensations, emotions and thoughts. Choosing a cognitive linguistic approach, Silvestre-López aims to establish what the analysis of 'mindfulness discourse' can reveal about the mental representations that underlie the mindfulness experience and practice. He encapsulates, from a linguistic perspective, the subjective experience associated with mindfulness by drawing on the linguistic production of the participants and practitioners of a series of mindfulness courses and identifying a series of conceptual metaphors and metonymic projections that are recurrently used in them. The study suggests that analysing this kind of discourse can lead to more effective mindfulness teaching procedures, including those of mindfulness-based psychotherapeutic programmes, and can become a rich source of data for further psychological experiments.

The contributions included in this volume, which are, in their majority, based on the analysis of empirical data, shed light on the understanding of the cognitive, textual, linguistic, ethical and discourse-specific features operating in medical discourse in professional, academic and popular settings. Some of the key genres in today's medical communication, such as those addressed to patients, scientific research and popular science articles and clinical cases, are examined in a wide variety of scenarios in order to provide new insights into the way medical professionals interact among each other, with patients and with society in general. The integrative, patient-oriented perspective that is adopted in the chapters dealing with the analysis of medical communication with patients reveals the way the medical profession as well as society (in particular the media) shape patients' understanding, knowledge and feelings about their illness. The fact that the training of medical professionals is the object of several contributions in this volume shows an awareness of the need to train professionals who are capable of engaging in a balanced and dynamic dialogue with patients.

As this volume shows, a societal approach to the language of medicine highlights the existence of a remarkable diversity of perspectives, issues and methods in this area, making it worth investigating. In fact, the relevance of language in medical practice is undeniable, as is the fact that its agents, mainly (but not only) practitioners and patients, can mutually benefit if the grounds for a successful interaction among them are correctly set. Interaction, communication and intelligibility are paramount for medical practice to run smoothly and for medical discourse to evolve and adapt to what society expects and demands. Despite its inherent complexity, attempts to better understand and improve medicine-related communication show that linguistic knowledge can be harnessed for science and that different epistemic domains can (and should) be intertwined to adapt to our rapidly changing world.

This book thus epitomises the richness of approaching science from a humanist perspective which merges language and science, medicine and society. The multidisciplinary analyses presented in this volume highlight the varied and complementary dimensions and perspectives within the language of medicine: ethical issues, comparative aspects of oral and written modes, metaphorical usage and function, teaching dimensions and implications, genre-related features, cultural and conceptual implications and psychology-related aspects such as mental representations within the framework of mindfulness. All the chapters show that approaching and understanding medicine from a more communicative, human and integrative perspective is one of the key challenges of current practitioners and scholars, and studies like this one are an important step in the right direction. Medical discourse should, thus, not be studied in isolation but in its true environment: society.

The language of medicine is a language by and for people, serving to articulate specialised knowledge, with either patients or practitioners as main agents, but also for translators, mediators, nurses and alternative therapy instructors. As such, it is the necessary means for epistemological transmission and cognitive evolution, but also for guaranteeing a crucial aspect of everybody's life: health.

This volume combines sociological and linguistic research applied to the medical field, showing the benefits derived from merging humanistic and scientific knowledge, since this approach creates synergies that can be highly beneficial for successful medical communication. All in all, the present volume is a very illustrative example of how linguists and translation specialists are building bridges between communication and medicine, in the same way that today's medicine is making efforts to build bridges between the two protagonists of medical discourse: professionals and patients.

References

Bowles, H. (2006) Conversation analysis and health communication: Updating a developing relationship. In M. Gotti and F. Salager-Meyer (eds) *Advances in Medical Discourse Analysis: Oral and Written Contexts* (pp. 43–64). Bern/Oxford: Peter Lang.

Candlin, S. (2006) Constructing knowledge, understanding and meaning between patients and nurses. In M. Gotti and F. Salager-Meyer (eds) *Advances in Medical Discourse Analysis: Oral and Written Contexts* (pp. 65–86). Bern/Oxford: Peter Lang.

Cordella, M. (2004) *The Dynamic Consultation. A Discourse Analytical Study of Doctor–Patient Communication*. Amsterdam/Philadelphia, PA: John Benjamins.

Gale, N.K. and McHale, J.V. (eds) (2015) *Routledge Handbook of Complementary and Alternative Medicine: Perspectives From Social Science and Law*. Abingdon/New York: Routledge.

García Izquierdo, I. and Montalt, V. (2013) Equigeneric and intergeneric translation in patient-centred care. *Hermes, Journal of Language and Communication in Business* 51, 39–51.

Gotti, M. (2014) Reformulation and recontextualization in popularization discourse. *IBÉRICA* 27, 15–34.

Gotti, M. and Salager-Meyer, F. (eds) (2006) *Advances in Medical Discourse Analysis: Oral and Written Contexts*. Bern/Oxford: Peter Lang.

Montalt, V. and Shuttleworth, M. (eds) (2012) Translation and knowledge mediation in medical and healthcare settings. *Linguistica Antverpiensia* 11, 9–29.

Pilegaard, M. (2007) Review of Marurizio Gotti and Françoise Salager-Meyer: *Advances in Medical Discourse Analysis: Oral and Written Contexts. LSP and Professional Communication* 7 (2), 113–118.

Salager-Meyer, F., Alcaraz Ariza, M.A., Pabón, M. and Zambrano, N. (2006) Paying one's intellectual debt: Acknowledgements in scientific/conventional and complementary/alternative medical research. In M. Gotti and F. Salager-Meyer (eds) *Advances in Medical Discourse Analysis: Oral and Written Contexts* (pp. 407–430). Bern/Oxford: Peter Lang.

Sarangi, S. (2012) Towards a communicative mentality in medical and healthcare practice. In K. Anna-Malin, M. Landqvist and H. Rehnberg (eds) *Med språket som arbetsredskap: Sju studier av kommunikation i vården* (pp. 13–34). Stockholm: Södertörns Högskola. (Modified and updated version of the inaugural editorial published as: Sarangi, S. [2004] Towards a communicative mentality in medical and healthcare practice. *Communication & Medicine* 1 (1), 1–11.)

Sharma, U. (2000) Medical pluralism and the future of CAM. In M. Kellner, B. Wellman, B. Pescosolido and M. Saks (eds) *Complementary and Alternative Medicine. Challenge and Change* (pp. 211–222). Abingdon/New York: Routledge.

Weingart, P. (2002) The moment of truth for science: The consequences of the 'knowledge society' for society and science. *EMBO Reports* 3 (8), 703–706.

2 Variations in Medical Discourse for Academic Purposes

Maurizio Gotti

This chapter investigates significant variations in medical discourse used for academic purposes, exploring the complex nature of its realisations. Indeed, in the last few years, medical discourse used for academic purposes has shown important variations deriving from a host of factors, such as cultural aspects, community membership, professional expertise and generic conventions. Moreover, a few research projects have pointed out differentiations in the behaviour of medical writers compared to that of members of other disciplinary fields. After a brief presentation of the evolution of medical discourse in academic contexts and the consolidation of the main medical text genres, the chapter will analyse the principal results of these previous studies.

The main part of the chapter will be devoted to the analysis of some significant data originating from a research project carried out by CERLIS, the research centre on specialised discourse based at the University of Bergamo. In this project, special attention has been given to the relationship between socioculturally oriented identity factors and textual variation in English specialised discourse, focusing in particular on the identification of identity traits typical of medical English compared to other branches of learning.

The data presented here show that the realisation of medical discourse in academic settings presents great variations in its generic textualisations. One of the key factors of this divergent verbal behaviour is certainly the affiliation of writers to different cultures (whether professional, ideological or ethnic-geographic); this does not only affect the medical discourse community's thinking and internal relationships but also the rhetorical 'positioning' of its participants. Moreover, the studies reported here also reflect the considerable challenges and opportunities that confront medical scholars seeking to achieve a delicate balance between their willingness to adhere to the norms and conventions of their professional community and the desire to express individual values and identity traits.

The Evolution of Medical Discourse in Academic Contexts

Medicine, as it is practised nowadays, developed largely in the 17th, 18th and 19th centuries. Scientific medicine (so called in opposition to complementary/alternative medicine referred to as 'unscientific' or unorthodox) is based on testable and replicable results published in research papers, review articles and meta-analyses. Evidence-based medicine has replaced the early medical traditions which were mainly based on the scholastic approach according to which the claims of prominent personalities were not to be discussed; they were, on the contrary, adopted as absolute truth (cf. Taavitsainen & Pahta, 2004). Before the 17th century, the doctrines of the ancient world dominated the theory and practice of Western medicine. Galenism, for example, taught that diseases resulted from an imbalance in the 'four humours', and that treatment with bloodletting and purging would re-establish equilibrium. This period was very important for the development of English medical discourse, as these centuries marked a remarkable increase in the use of the vernacular for medical and scientific writing. Indeed, at the beginning of this period, Latin still had a dominant role. At the end of this period, English prevailed, and the process of vernacularisation can be described as largely completed by 1700, when we can find a full range of sophisticated university treatises on medicine in English where Latin played little or no role. Indeed, of the 238 medical books published in the years 1640–1660, 207 were in English (Webster, 1974: 267).

Great epistemological and methodological developments took place in that period, both in medicine and surgery: old scholastic thinking began to be replaced by new patterns of thought and new methodologies based on observation and interpretation of physical phenomena (cf. Hunter, 1989; Jardine, 1999; Shapiro, 2000; Vickers, 1987). These developments determined the need for corresponding changes both in the ways of communicating the new discoveries attained by means of innovative procedures and apparatus, and in the expressive tools to be used to describe and argue about the new phenomena observed and analysed. The evolution of the methods adopted in the study of medicine and the development of new medical and surgical procedures implied a change not only in the approach to the interpretation of the issues analysed, but also in the way in which phenomena ought to be described and opinions expressed. The realisation that the English language was inadequate for the needs of expression of men of science led to its gradual amelioration, both from a quantitative and a qualitative point of view. British scientists made great efforts to increase the number of specialised terms and to improve the exactness of their meanings (cf. Gotti, 2011: 153–169). Also from the textual point of view, there was a great development in this period; the early printed works mainly consisted of translations of treatises and new compositions of general guides to health and handbooks of medical instructions, often including accounts of illustrative and typical cases (Bennett, 1969). The 18th century, instead, showed a greater variety of genres, with the addition of new forms such as anatomical observations, book reviews (BRs), journal articles (Lefanu, 1937) and experimental essays (Gotti, 2001).

The great developments in medical research and practice are well reflected in the growing number of medical journals published annually worldwide and of non-medical journals devoted to the (linguistic, sociolinguistic, socio-historical, etc.) study of medical discourse. Every year, over 5 million medical papers in several different languages are published by about 25,000 medical journals (Cooter, 2000). This hyperinflation of information is mostly due to the fact that each discipline is subject to a subdivision every 10 years, which in turn leads to the creation of new specialised journals (Régent, 2000). If we add to this figure the 500 or so journals in nursing and dentistry and the non-medical journals dealing with medical issues and discourse, the final figure is 10 million health-related papers published each year. Not only 'conventional' but also unconventional medical journals (Brodin & Danell, 2005) are steadily on the increase. Indeed, complementary and alternative medical therapies (CAM) have attracted increased national attention from the media, the medical community, government agencies and the public (see Salager-Meyer *et al.*, 2006). Surveys performed in the USA and elsewhere suggest that CAM is popular throughout the industrialised world (Eisenberg *et al.*, 1998; Goldbeck-Wood *et al.*, 1996), and the number of CAM papers published both in CAM journals and in conventional medical journals such as *JAMA*, *BMJ* and the *Annals of Internal Medicine*, is growing at a very fast rate (Brodin & Danell, 2005).

Medical Written Genres in Academic Contexts

The evolution of medical discourse in academic contexts has promoted the rise and consolidation of different text genres, which have acquired well-established norms. Indeed, there is a close link between a type of medical text and its structure, which in turn implies a number of correlations between the conceptual, rhetorical and linguistic features that characterise the text itself. Genre not only provides a conventional framework but also affects all other textual features and constrains their conceptual and rhetorical development. With time, several text types have arisen – some derived from genres common in general language, others crafted specifically to meet the needs of specialists. Through training and professional engagement, specialists learn to follow given norms and patterns in each type of text; the conventional use of genres also produces certain expectations among their audience, and whenever the rules are broken, a text is misunderstood or rejected. Discourse analysts have discovered the importance of the concept of genre not only to get a better understanding of the linguistic characteristics of texts, but also of the macrostructure of these texts, which appears to be organised according to genre expectations and conventions rooted in the sociocultural context. This is the reason why in recent years genre theory has taken a more serious look at context in a much broader sense, paying particular attention to text/context interactions focusing not simply on the form and content of genres, but more importantly on how genres are constructed, interpreted, used and exploited in the achievement of specific goals in highly specialised contexts. Indeed, communicative situations combine several contextual factors, making it difficult to attribute a given linguistic peculiarity to a single originating factor. This awareness has led scholars to group together the contextual factors capable of identifying the parameters which distinguish different genres within a specialised language.

Several studies have pointed out that, although different texts have specific generic characteristics (Bhatia, 1993, 2004; Swales, 1990, 2004), they allow writers a certain degree of flexibility. At the same time, textual genres themselves are not stable but highly dynamic and closely related to their socio-professional contexts (Berkenkotter *et al.*, 2012; Bhatia & Gotti, 2006). Indeed, genres vary according to several factors, the main ones being the communicative purposes they aim to fulfil, the settings or contexts in which they are employed, the communicative events or activities they are associated with, the professional relationships existing between the people taking part in such activities or events and the background knowledge of each participant. For example, depending upon their degree of innovativeness, medical genres differ as follows: texts which are meant to convey original information and innovative data belong to the primary genres, which include research papers, case reports and editorials; texts that rely on them belong to the secondary genre category, such as review articles, BRs and pedagogical texts (Swales, 2004). Medical texts also differ according to the degree of specialised knowledge of their readership: in this case texts will be divided into two main categories: professional and popular. Professional texts are aimed at medical professionals (researchers, practitioners and students of medicine), whereas popular texts are targeted at the general readership. Texts aimed at professionals are written by medical professionals, while the writers of popular texts include both medical professionals and non-professionals, such as popularisers or journalists.

Table 2.1 Medical written genres, subdivided on the basis of their audience design

Professional texts	*Popular texts*
Research papers	Newspaper/magazine articles
Case reports	Guidebook samples
Editorials	Informative material ...
Review articles	
Book reviews	
Pedagogic texts ...	

The two criteria illustrated above may be combined and exemplified in Table 2.1.

A third classification can be obtained if taking into consideration the communicative function of the texts and their writer's intention. In this case, texts may be divided into argumentative, directive and expository genres (Vihla, 1999). Argumentative genres are meant to convince the readers, directive ones are those that provide advice on how to act while expository genres have the purpose of explaining or describing. This tripartite categorisation of genres reflects the complex and varied field of application of medicine: on the one hand, medicine belongs to the world of science as it is the site where new scientific knowledge is constructed through hypotheses and tested through reliable methods. In this field of medical research, experimentation can be considered the main activity, and argumentative texts the main product, as they are meant to convince other medical professionals of the validity of the results achieved. Directive and expository genres, on the other hand, relate to the practical side of medicine, as the function of the former is to provide recommendations on the best practices to professionals (e.g. handbooks and clinical manuals) and advice to non-professionals (e.g. guidebooks), while the latter are meant to disseminate scientific background knowledge to members of the in-group (e.g. medical textbooks) and the out-group (e.g. popularising articles and informative material). The complexity of the medical field and its genres are exemplified in Table 2.2.

Table 2.2 Three-dimensional genre classification based on audience design, genre and communicative function

	Argumentative	*Directive*	*Expository*
Professional	Research articles	Handbook samples	Medical textbooks
	Editorials	Clinical manuals	
Popular		Guidebook samples	Popularising articles
			Informative material

Source: Adapted from Pahta (2006: 362).

Intercultural Variation in Medical Written Genres

In recent years, the great increase in cooperation and collaboration at an international level has accelerated the globalisation of sociocultural and communicative practices. This globalising process has strongly favoured English, which over the last century or so has become the preferred medium for international communication in many contexts. The strict English-medium policies adopted by many academic publications and book series have aroused non-English speakers' awareness that the increasing use of this language in publishing and higher education might greatly reduce the role of national languages for academic purposes. Indeed, as there is a tendency of scholars to publish what they consider to be their best work in English so as to reach a wider audience (cf. among others, Bolton & Kuteeva, 2012; Gunnarsson, 2000, for Sweden; Yakhontova, 2001, for Ukraine; Salager-Meyer *et al.*, 2003, for Latin America; Giannoni, 2008, for Italy; Kachru, 2009, for Asia; Brock-Utne, 2001, for the Nordic Countries; and Ferguson *et al.*, 2011, for Spain), non-English-medium publications are often relegated to the status of local scholarly products providing only a marginal contribution to the mainstream because they are unable to disseminate knowledge through a global lingua franca. For some scholars (cf. Canagarajah, 2002; Kandiah, 2005), the considerable success of English in the world of academic research poses a threat not only to the survival and productivity of other languages but also for researchers from non-English-speaking cultures, whose perception of specialised discourse inevitably diverges from the dominant Anglo-American model(s). In this sense, Mauranen (1993) claims that weaker academic discourses deserve attention and protection on a par with vanishing ecosystems, while Swales (1997) describes English as a tyrant in the field.

This spread of English has had relevant ideological and ethical implications (Pérez-Llantada, 2012): as globalising trends commonly rely on covert strategies meant to reduce participants' specificities, they hybridise local identities in favour of Anglocentric textual models. Globalisation thus offers a topical illustration of the interaction between linguistic and cultural factors in the construction of discourse, both within specialised domains and in wider contexts (Candlin & Gotti, 2004, 2007). As language is strictly linked to the setting in which it is used, cultural elements may operate as key contextual constraints, influencing both the level of discursive organisation and its range of realisations (Hyland, 2011). Being associated with communities linked to local as well as international conventions, medical discourse has provided fertile ground for the analysis of intercultural variation, both at a textual level and in the communicative strategies embedded in its textualisations. Several research projects have investigated identity-forming features linked to 'local' or disciplinary cultures, as communicated through English in various academic domains by native (NSs) and non-native speakers (NNSs). Three recent projects on this issue are the KIAP Project (Cultural Identity in Academic Prose, http://www.uib.no/kiap/), carried out by the University of Bergen, Norway; the SERAC Project (Spanish/English Research Article Corpus), conducted at the University of Zaragoza (www.interlae.com); and the Identity and Culture in Academic Discourse Project, carried out by CERLIS, the research centre on specialised discourse based at the University of Bergamo (www.unibg.it/cerlis). By exploring the international perspective suggested by major social and academic actors, they have evaluated how far international audiences in key intercultural domains adopt textual reconfigurations that simplify, distort or even remove non-congruent institutional and cultural traits, while enhancing the identities of specific social and professional communities.

The KIAP Project, for example, has carried out a comparative analysis of medical research articles (RAs) with those of two other disciplines: economics and linguistics. In particular, Fløttum (2006) compared articles written in three different languages: English, French and Norwegian, in order to establish whether cultural identities may be identified in academic prose, and, if so, whether these identities are language- or discipline-specific in nature. As regards the comparison of medical RAs with those of the other two disciplines investigated, her analysis indicated that medical RAs are normally multi-authored, while most of the articles in the other two disciplines are single-authored, particularly in linguistics as shown by the following ratios (the first figure represents single-authored articles): linguistics: 131/19; economics: 87/63; medicine: 15/135. Moreover, as regards author presence, medical authors are not very visible in their texts, as compared to their economist and linguist peers. They 'hide' behind passive constructions and impersonal formulations of different kinds. Observations 'present themselves' to a larger extent than in economics and linguistics articles.

Another interesting difference concerns the frequency with which authors refer to (parts of) the text itself, with metatextual expressions with which the author guides the readers through the article itself (as *in this article*) or explains what will be done and where (e.g. *in section 4 we analyse* ...). The results of Fløttum's analysis indicate very clearly that this feature is more or less absent in medical articles, while it is present in the other two disciplines particularly in linguistics articles (with 1230 occurrences against only 47 in medical articles). Moreover, in medical articles, Fløttum did not find much direct argumentation of the type *we argue* or *in this article we have shown*. This does not mean that medical researchers do not argue. Argumentation is not only to be found in personal constructions introduced by personal pronouns. The strategies used by medical authors to convince their readers are commonly realised by the presentation of facts or observations in 'neutral' utterances which at first glance appear as both objective and deprived of personal traces.

Another aspect investigated is the frequency of bibliographical references. Fløttum's study indicates that references in a medical article are listed at the end and are indicated by numbers in the body of the text. In economics and linguistics, instead, references are typically introduced (in different ways) in the text itself. As regards the number of references referred to (whether introduced by number or by author name+year of publication), she found that medical authors use more references than economists and linguists. When looking at how authors of cited articles are 'given the floor', a similar interesting differentiation emerges: cited linguists are allowed to *argue* and to *claim* something while cited medical authors (and also to a large extent cited economists) are typically only allowed to *find* or to *show* results and observations.

Another issue investigated was how authors present their final results, in particular how explicitly they present them. The analysis showed that the word *results* with the meaning 'final results' is more or less absent in linguistics articles, but is quite frequent in medical and especially in economics articles. However, when *results* is used to refer to 'final results', the context is typically a 'neutral' one, with few or no colouring, personal or evaluative elements:

(1) The results of this study demonstrate a number of such potential mediators. (Fløttum, 2006: 262)

On examining the verbs combined with first-person pronouns, Fløttum has found that these verbs indicate that the authors assume various roles when referring to themselves by the pronoun *we*. Linguists play at least three different roles, i.e. arguers (*we argue*), writers or readers' guide (*in section 3 we will present*) and researchers (*we analyse, we find*). Economists generally take on only the researcher or the writer roles, while medical authors stick to the researcher role. A further illustration of this is that the three most frequent verbs combined with *we* in the multi-author articles studied in KIAP are *find, assume, use* in economics, *find, argue, see* in linguistics, *find, use, examine* in medicine. This difference may be due to epistemological reasons: medical research is more cumulative and need not discuss basic conceptual systems in the same way as linguistics often does. Moreover, in medicine, the reported research is typically presented as completed when the writing of the article starts; in linguistics, the research is often presented as if it is part of the writing process itself. Furthermore, by adhering strictly to the introduction, methods, results and discussion (IMRAD) article structure, medical authors need not guide the reader or make explicit transitions from one section to another in the same way as linguists and economists do in their often much more heterogeneously structured articles.

In general, Fløttum's findings show that for cultural identities, discipline has greater influence than language. This means that, for example, there are more similarities between Norwegian and French medical articles than between Norwegian medical and linguistic articles. Statistically both discipline and language have an effect on the frequency of all the six main phenomena studied. However, for most of them, discipline seems to be more important than language.

The CERLIS Project

In the CERLIS Project special attention has been given to the relationship between socioculturally oriented identity factors and textual variation in English academic discourse, focusing in particular on the detection of identity traits typical of different branches of learning. Within such domains, we have investigated to what extent the cultural allegiance of (native or non-native) anglophone discourse communities to their linguistic, professional, social or national reference groups is affected by the use of English as a lingua franca of international communication. As corpora constitute a remarkable tool for the study of discourse, a specific corpus (Corpus of Academic Discourse, or CADIS)[1] was assembled as the core and foundation of this line of research.

Because of our interest in intercultural communication, our research unit selected a range of texts produced by scholars and academic institutions in different parts of the world. To identify textual variants arising from the use of English as a native language or lingua franca of science, and to contrast them with those written in Italian by NSs, we devised a corpus formed by academic texts in English and Italian. Besides including two languages, CADIS represents four different disciplinary areas: applied linguistics, economics, law and medicine. For each disciplinary area, four different genres were considered: RAs, abstracts, BRs and editorials. To allow also for diachronic variation in academic discourse over the last 30 years, the texts were divided into two different time groups: 1980–1999 and 2000–2011. The original structure of the corpus is shown in Table 2.3.

Including all language groups – NSs and NNSs of English, and NSs of Italian – a total of 2738 texts (from 635 to 739 per disciplinary area) – have been inserted in the corpus. At present, the corpus includes over 12 million words.

Table 2.3 The structure of CADIS

Disciplinary area	*No. of articles*	*No. of abstracts*	*No. of book reviews*	*No. of editorials*
Applied linguistics	160	166	172	137
1980–1999: ENG	32	50	40	20
1980–1999: ITA	6	6	5	4
2000–2011: ENG	112	100	110	110
2000–2011: ITA	10	10	17	3
Economics	174	162	150	166
1980–1999: ENG	50	50	50	39
1980–1999: ITA	6	6	–	13
2000–2011: ENG	112	100	100	103
2000–2011: ITA	15	5	4	10
Law	226	187	172	127
1980–1999: ENG	68	50	60	8
1980–1999: ITA	14	14	–	2
2000–2011: ENG	94	100	100	113
2000–2011: ITA	50	23	12	4
Medicine	222	210	119	188
1980–1999: ENG	40	40	13	50
1980–1999: ITA	10	11	1	4
2000–2011: ENG	117	105	100	123
2000–2011: ITA	55	55	5	11
Total	782	725	613	618

Textual variations in journal editorials

Our research project has dealt with identity traits across languages and cultures, as the use of a given language affects the writing of a scholar, especially when it is not his or her native language. This is particularly evident in the case of English, whose recurrent use by NNSs requires a degree of adaptation of their thought patterns and expressive habits. These issues have been dealt with by various members of the CERLIS team. Giannoni (2012), for example, has investigated local vs global identities in medical editorials (MEDs). His analysis of Anglo-American journals, English-medium Italian journals and standard Italian journals suggests the considerable extent of intradisciplinary variation, both within and across languages/cultures. The data investigated thus allow for the observation of the writing behaviour of three different kinds of scholars: native speaker English (NEng), non-native (i.e. Italian) English (ItEng) and native speaker Italian (NIt).[2] Since (MEDs) are signed by only one or two authors, native-speaker status is relatively easy to determine, based on the author's name and affiliation.

Table 2.4 Average size of texts by section

	Length (tokens)	*Range*	*Tokens/paragraph*
NEng	1046	619–1809	125
ItEng	1882	609–3637	113
NIt	2429	1154–5222	87

A quantitative overview of the material (Table 2.4) shows interesting differences between the three sections in terms of average length, with NEng texts less than half the size of their NIt counterparts and ItEng somewhere in between. On the other hand, discourse complexity, as measured by average paragraph length, is greatest in NEng (44% higher than NIt). These figures suggest that while Italian MEDs are lengthier than their native English counterparts, they organise the discourse into far shorter units. For both parameters, the ItEng group occupies the middle ground between the two.

Giannoni's analysis shows that editorialists employ three types of MEDs, whose prominence and microlinguistic traits vary across the corpus:

- *Advice* editorials are authoritative reviews of medical issues providing guidance for practitioners.
- *Comment editorials* are opinionated interpretations of developments affecting the medical community, with recommendations for action.
- *Message editorials* reinforce the journal's relationship with its readers, keeping them informed of its initiatives and developments.

While the orientation of the first subgenre is mainly teleological – i.e. driven by the need to shape medical practice – the second is evaluative and the third is phatic. A rough indication of the respective weight of these subgenres across the corpus is given in Table 2.5, which includes a fourth column, due to the presence in NIt of three spurious text types presented as *editoriale* (namely a review article, an essay and a conference talk). Interestingly, the three subgenres are documented across the corpus, with the sole exception of comment editorials. These are indeed the most variable subgroup, accounting for 80% of texts in NEng but none in ItEng. On the other hand, advice editorials are used far less, proportionally speaking, in NEng (10%) than in the two groups authored by Italians.

Table 2.5 Proportion of MED subgenres across the corpus sample

	Advice (%)	*Comment (%)*	*Message (%)*	*Other (%)*
NEng	10	80	10	–
ItEng	60	–	40	–
NIt	50	10	10	30

These data warrant the hypothesis that Italian editorialists: (a) are less likely to comment on current affairs and issues of a (non-)medical nature, whether writing in their first language or in English; and (b) understand the 'editorial' not only as a genre but also (in NIt) as a slot for publishing other genres that deserve editorial sanction. Moreover, unlike their NEng counterparts, Italian writers are likely to incorporate references into their own work – a self-promotional strategy observed in all the ItEng texts and in 40% of the NIt sample. Italian scholars appear therefore to be freer in their use of the MED genre, with no clear-cut distinction between the role of editorialist (knowledge validation) and that of researcher (knowledge construction). The high rate of self-citations in ItEng indicates that the two functions are particularly blurred when editorialists address an international audience through the medium of English.

One notable difference between the NEng texts (e.g. Quotation 2) and the other two groups (e.g. Quotations 3 and 4) is (with only one exception) the absence among the latter of direct appeals to the medical community. When a course of action is advocated, as in (4), its wording is both impersonal and indirect. Viewed contrastively, this difference may reflect the more tentative orientation of NIt MEDs (rhetorical interference) but also – more intriguingly – greater interpersonal distance in the ItEng sample, where local (Italian) academics address a global community of which they are, linguistically speaking, only peripheral members.

(2) We still have hurdles of ethics, immunology and biology to conquer, and until we do, we must remain on guard against donor scotoma. (NEng, MEED494)
(3) Therefore, we believe that right insula activation has a significant role in the perception of chest pain in syndrome X (the insula is known to receive cardiopulmonary inputs). (ItEng, MEED511)
(4) Tale strategia può contribuire a ridurre in maniera significativa il rischio di reazioni avverse a farmaci idrosolubili e i costi sanitari ad esse correlati [This strategy may help to significantly reduce the risk of adverse reactions to hydrosoluble drugs and their associated healthcare costs]. (NIt, MEED916)

Comment editorials were the second most common type of MED but also that with the greatest range of variation across the corpus, accounting for 80% of NEng, 10% of NIt and none of the ItEng texts. Interestingly, all the NEng instances come from the oldest, most firmly established publication in the corpus (*Journal of Clinical Investigation*). This suggests that critical commentaries are more likely to originate from Anglo-American contexts, where the editorial stance of certain journals allows a high level of 'militancy'.

The purpose of message editorials is essentially phatic, insofar as they seek to forge/maintain a strong relationship with the readership by keeping it informed of editorial decisions and policies. Consequently, editorialists act here in an institutional as well as an individual capacity. Altogether, this was the least common MED subgenre observed in the corpus, accounting for only 10% of texts in NEng and NIt. The figure rises to 40% in the ItEng group – which suggests that the effort to engage readers overtly is greatest for English-medium publications originating from the periphery. In ItEng, however, message editorials are always meta-texts introducing/promoting the journal's advice editorials. The different use of message editorials across the CADIS sample is clearly observable in their macrostructure. The two texts in NEng/NIt are essentially unstructured narratives bringing to the attention of readers important developments in the journal's life (and/or that of its affiliates). Such MEDs span events in the past, present and near future, as shown by the following excerpts:

(5) The wind of change is in the air again. *The British Journal of Plastic Surgery* is a great and almost a venerable title, but it seems that BJPS can never stand still. [...] Many of our readers are discovering the benefits of Science Direct, which carries the full text of BJPS from the very first issue, available on line and fully searchable through hypertext links. [...] Now, from January 1st 2006, our journal will become JPRAS, *The Journal of Plastic, Reconstructive and Aesthetic Surgery*, and will be published every month. (NEng, MEED498)

(6) Con questo numero, l'*Italian Heart Journal* diviene organo di stampa anchedella Società Italiana di Chirurgia Cardiaca. [...] È ormai nei fatti della nostra attività clinica quotidiana il sempre più stretto legame e la proficua integrazione di competenze tra specialisti cardiologi e cardiochirurghi. [...] L'*Italian Heart Journal*avrà un compito importanteed impegnativo nel sostenere le sempre più numeroseiniziative che le Società di settore stanno cercando diportare avanti. [With this issue the *Italian Heart Journal* becomes an official publication of the Italian Heart Surgery Society. [...] Our daily clinical practice already bears witness to the ever closer link and fruitful integration of competences between heart specialists and heart surgeons. [...] *The Italian Heart Journal* will face the important and challenging task of supporting the increasing number of initiatives that medical societies are attempting to conduct.] (NIt, MEED907)

Giannoni's analysis thus shows that, as a consequence of the composite generic profile of the medical editorials analysed and of the coexistence of no less than three distinct subgenres (Advice, Comment, Message),

Table 2.6 Generic profile of medical editorials

Subgenre	*Voice*	*Target*
Advice	Expert	Disciplinary knowledge
Comment	Journal	World
Message	Editor	Journal and editor

editorialists are keen to adapt their voice to the specific communicative purpose text, taking on a different identity and evaluating a different target, as summarised in Table 2.6.

Moreover, the multilingual and multicultural environment in which scholars are working within a globalised context implies that editorialists are faced with the challenge of reconciling two 'small cultures' (their local academic community and linguacultural affiliation) with a 'large culture' (the discipline as a global, translinguistic community). The easy option is to concentrate on the latter, forgetting that it can only emerge through a process of negotiation involving the former. Italian scholars appear to be avoiding this risk and draft English editorials that do not merely incorporate elements of the NEng/NIt repertoire but do so in innovative and at times creative ways.

Textual variations in book reviews

In her analysis of BRs written in English and Italian by native (NSs) and non-native speakers (NNSs), D'Angelo (2012) has investigated how reviewers of different nationalities, within the disciplines of applied linguistics, economics, law and medicine, express positive and negative appraisals (respectively PAs and NAs) of their peers' work. The comparison of the English and Italian sections of the corpus has shown that in all the disciplines considered in the study, BRs written in English are generally much longer than BRs written in Italian (cf. Table 2.7). One factor of a quantitative nature could account for the greater variation in length

Table 2.7 Corpus size

	English			*Italian*		
	Running words in subcorpus	*%*	*Average length of BR*	*Running words in subcorpus*	*%*	*Average length of BR*
Applied linguistics	48,521	24.7	1617.3	4,842	19.8	372.4
Economics	36,173	18.4	1205.7	6,074	24.8	467.2
Law	89,322	45.6	2977.4	3,635	14.8	279.6
Medicine	22,016	11.3	733.8	9,964	40.6	766.4
Total	196,032			24,515		

Table 2.8 Running words in BRs written in English by NS and NNS

		Average length of English BRs	%
Applied linguistics	NS	1568.4	12.3
	NNS	1666.2	12.9
Economics	NS	1016	7.9
	NNS	1397	10.8
Law	NS	2843.2	22
	NNS	2945.5	22.9
Medicine	NS	652	5
	NNS	790	6.2

observed in Italian and English BRs: in every discipline, different journals impose different word limits on BR writers. However, there seems to be different cultural norms and traditions when it comes to producing BRs for Italian journals. In the discipline of applied linguistics, economics and law, all of the Italian journals limited the amount of words (and therefore the space and depth) of BRs. The biggest difference in the average length of texts is found in the discipline of law, where Italian BRs are 10 times shorter than the English ones, and in the discipline of applied linguistics, where Italian BRs are four times shorter than the English ones. In medicine on the other hand, BRs are found to be of the same length, and therefore the 'cultural' trend of limiting the use and space of BRs does not seem to apply to this discipline.

If we concentrate on BRs written in English (Table 2.8), an interesting finding is that in all four disciplines considered, NNSs seem to produce slightly longer BRs than NSs.

Also Rowley-Jolivet and Carter-Thomas (2005: 45) found that clauses in NNS texts (RAs and paper presentations) are considerably longer than in NS texts, something accountable to the more frequent use of the passive form by NNSs than by NSs, which leads to the production of longer, more articulated sentences.

The investigation of different disciplines has shown that the use of PAs and NAs is surprisingly consistent: PAs are always used at least twice (if not three times) as often as NAs. What is interesting to note is that in law, English reviewers evaluate a book negatively much more frequently than in other disciplines (cf. Table 2.9). Reviewers in economics also use NAs frequently in comparison with other disciplines, whereas in medicine, they do so much more rarely. When we consider the use of appraisal in Italian, we cannot but notice that the only reviewers that try to reach a balance between positive and negative evaluations are the ones working in the field of economics (the numbers are 7.3 NAs vs 13 PAs). On the contrary, the authors who use NAs the least and are undeniably much more prone to positive peer reviewing, are the ones writing in law (2.8 occurrences of NAs vs 37.5 of PAs).

Table 2.9 Occurrences of NAs and PAs in different disciplines

		NA	*PA*
Applied linguistics	ENG	10.1	15
	ITA	7.7	28.9
Economics	ENG	12.8	22.6
	ITA	7.3	13
Law	ENG		
	NS		
	NNS	22.9	36.4
	ITA	2.8	37.5
Medicine	ENG	5.5	16.2
	ITA	4.4	27.3

Table 2.10 Occurrences of NAs and PAs in different disciplines, by NS and NNS

			NA	*PA*
Applied linguistics	ENG	NS	8.1	10.1
		NNS	4.9	6.7
Economics	ENG	NS	8	15.2
		NNS	4.7	7.3
Law	ENG	NS	11.3	16
		NNS	6.8	25
Medicine	ENG	NS	3.6	12.5
		NNS	1.8	3.6

If in every discipline we further differentiate between native and non-native reviewers, we notice that the use of NAs and PAs follows a clear pattern: every discipline considered sees NNSs consistently using almost twice as many PAs as NAs (cf. Table 2.10). These data further validate the hypothesis that NNSs, in every discipline, tend to use evaluation less frequently and, most of all, they tend to prefer evaluating positively rather than negatively.

Textual variations in research articles

Maci (2012) has compared the argumentative strategies employed in medical RAs written by NSs of English with those written by Italian NNSs of English in order to identify any cross-cultural differences in terms of argumentative devices employed by their authors. Analysing the *Discussion* section of 50 articles from two important journals of cardiology – the *Italian Heart Journal* (published in English) which, in 2006, changed its name to the *Journal of Cardiovascular Medicine*,[3] and the American journal *Circulation*

– she has identified several differences between the textual organisation of English medical RAs written by NSs and NNSs, which seem to be linked to their authors' linguistic and cultural identity. The main differences are rhetorically realised through hedges and other argumentative strategies, such as the use of connectives. Indeed, NSs of English tend to exploit more fully modality expressed by modal auxiliaries (such as *may, would*), verbs (such as *appear, suggest*) and adverbs (such as *likely*). The modal verb *may*, in particular, frequently appears in the NSs corpus, to such an extent that it can be regarded as a keyword with high keyness (*may* occupies position 15). This is not the case in the Italian NNSs subcorpus, where *may* occupies position 95.

The minimal use of hedges in the Italian NNSs subcorpus seems to be counterbalanced by other grammatical devices: whenever the outcome conforms to the expected results and is thus validated, Italian authors tend to interpret outcomes with the use of the present tense of such boosters as *confirm, find* and *show* rather than using hedging devices. If hedges are used, there is a preference for *might*, which may be perceived by NNSs as carrying a stronger connotation of probability than *may*, or *should*, employed whenever a suggestion about the correct scientific procedures and/or treatment is made. This occurs especially whenever the results do not confirm the initial hypothesis, or whenever there is a gap in the existing literature filled by the present research. In these cases, NNSs of English seem to prefer the use of hedges and modal expressions to indicate probable interpretations or possible implications.

The use of hedges is mitigated by the presence of supporting evidence provided by previous studies in the same field, with quotations employed so as to establish academic credibility. References are inserted as matter of fact, thus making them more certain and strengthening the case made. Results are therefore made meaningful because researchers refer to previous accounts of formal research. Furthermore, quotations are not listed as anonymous numbers; rather, they are *personified* by quoting the surname of the author(s) of previous studies.

A further differentiation can be seen in the use of connectives. There is a lower frequency of connectives in RAs written by NNSs of English, which seems to reflect the trend already established by Italian authors as far as the use of hedges is concerned: whenever the claim is confirmed and supported by scientific literature in the field, Italian researchers seem less keen on exploiting argumentative strategies, as, apparently, reference to the literature becomes the objective evidence supporting the author's reasoning.

Moreover, Italian authors seem to prefer the use of an *ipse dixit* strategy: whenever a claim finds confirmation in the existing literature, they tend to adopt rhetorical strategies less frequently because the established knowledge is deemed to be sufficient to confirm their hypothesis.

Variation in the use of metaphoric expressions

Giannoni (2010) has also investigated the use of metaphoric expressions in NS English RAs published in peer-reviewed journals from four domains (economics, law, medicine, linguistics). His analysis shows that evaluative metaphors vary considerably across disciplines in terms of source domain, connotations and polarisation, and that they are linked not only to disciplinary proclivities but also to a discipline's metaphoric identity. As shown by the weight of the top three metaphoric values in each domain (cf. Table 2.11), there is a relative degree of similarity as well as variation across disciplines in the choice of metaphorically evaluative lexis.

The most noticeable finding is the prevalence of *SIGNIFICANT* over all other values, especially in medicine and, to a lesser extent, in linguistics. It appears therefore that SIGNIFICANCE is a highly strategic aspect of research, especially in the latter two domains. However, a semantic distinction needs to be made between *SIGNIFICANT*='statistically valid' (i.e. *no significant differences in allele or genotype frequencies were found for the other six variants*) and *SIGNIFICANT*='meaningful' (i.e. *when an event has great significance or elicits negative emotional responses for an individual, he may display the topic's emotional load through vocal changes*). The relative weight of their two uses is shown in Table 2.12.

The most striking difference is observed in medicine, which appears to view SIGNIFICANCE only as a mathematical quality, carefully avoiding other interpretations of this metaphor. The statistically measurable dimension of research is emphasised also in economics (92%) and linguistics (85%). The opposite case applies to legal studies, where *SIGNIFICANT* is used

Table 2.11 Metaphoric values by domain

Domain	*Value*	*Frequency/10,000 words*
Linguistics	*SIGNIFICANT*	9.93
	CLEAR	5.99
	STRONG	4.16
Economics	*SIGNIFICANT*	6.58
	STRONG	5.96
	CONSISTENT	3.34
Law	*MANAGEABLE*	8.88
	CLEAR	7.80
	SIGNIFICANT	5.19
Medicine	*SIGNIFICANT*	16.22
	CONSISTENT	6.84
	MANAGEABLE	4.02

Source: From Giannoni (2010: 285).

Table 2.12 Semantic distribution of *SIGNIFICANT*

	LING	*ECO*	*LAW*	*MED*
'Statistically valid'	8.40 (85%)	6.06 (92%)	0.11 (2%)	16.22 (100%)
'Meaningful'	1.53 (15%)	0.52 (8%)	5.08 (98%)	–
Total	9.93	6.58	5.19	16.22

Source: From Giannoni (2010: 287).

almost exclusively (98%) in an overtly subjective, non-statistical sense arising from jurisprudence and legal interpretation. On the other hand, the concern for CLARITY is most prominent in law and linguistics, which, unlike their counterparts, rely more heavily on speculative knowledge than experimental evidence. Economics and linguistics attribute particular importance to STRENGTH, relating almost exclusively to experimental data and their interpretation (*strong correlation/assumption/prediction/evidence/effects*). The value of MANAGEABILITY is most prominent in law and common in medicine but extremely rare in the other domains, while CONSISTENCY is emphasised especially in medicine and economics, when discussing data or experimental results.

Conclusion

As shown by the data analysed in this chapter, the realisation of medical discourse in academic settings presents great variations in its various generic textualisations. One of the key factors of this divergent verbal behaviour is certainly the affiliation of writers to various cultures (whether professional, ideological or ethnic-geographic); this not only affects the medical discourse community's thinking and internal relationships but also the rhetorical 'positioning' of its participants. Moreover, the studies reported here reflect the considerable challenges and opportunities that confront medical scholars seeking to achieve a delicate balance between their willingness to adhere to the norms and conventions of their professional community and the desire to express individual values and identity traits. Such factors have been found to interact, producing textual realisations characterised by variant forms that often betray their dependence on local traits and traditions.

Notes

(1) A breakdown of the corpus is available online at www.unibg.it/cerlis.

(2) The journals investigated are as follows: *British Journal of Plastic Surgery* and the US-based *Journal of Clinical Investigation* for NEng; English editorials from two bilingual journals, the *Italian Heart Journal* and *Epidemiologia e Psichiatria Sociale*, for ItEng; the *Giornale Italiano di Cardiologia* and *Recenti Progressi in Medicina* for NIt.

(3) Since, in Italy, Italian journals, despite their in-depth analyses, are regarded as second-class research tools by the local medical community, and since medical journals are regarded as being serious only if they are published in English, either in the UK or in the US, the Italian scientific board of the *Italian Heart Journal* decided to conceal the Italian-like quality of the journal by assigning it an English name (*Journal of Cardiovascular Medicine*) and an American publisher, while maintaining an Italian editorial and scientific board.

References

Bennett, H.S. (1969) *English Books and Readers 1475–1557*. Cambridge: Cambridge University Press.

Berkenkotter, C., Bhatia, V.J. and Gotti, M. (eds) (2012) *Insights into Academic Genres*. Bern: Peter Lang.

Bhatia, V.K. (1993) *Analysing Genre: Language Use in Professional Settings*. London: Longman.

Bhatia, V.K. (2004) *Worlds of Written Discourse: A Genre-Based View*. London: Continuum.

Bhatia, V.J. and Gotti, M. (eds) (2006) *Explorations in Specialized Genres*. Bern: Peter Lang.

Bolton, K. and Kuteeva, M. (2012) English as an academic language at a Swedish University: Parallel language use and the 'threat' of English. *Journal of Multilingual and Multicultural Development* 33/5, 429–447.

Brock-Utne, B. (2001) The growth of English for academic communication in the Nordic countries. *International Review of Education* 47, 221–233.

Brodin, J.A. and Danell, R. (2005) Spiritualised medicine? A bibliometric study of complementary and alternative medicine (CAM). Paper delivered at the 4th EASST Conference, Paris, August.

Canagarajah, S. (2002) *A Geopolitics of Academic Writing*. Pittsburgh, PA: University of Pittsburgh Press.

Candlin, C. and Gotti, M. (eds) (2004) *Intercultural Discourse in Domain-Specific English*. Special issue of *Textus* 17/1.

Candlin, C. and Gotti, M. (eds) (2007) *Intercultural Aspects of Specialized Communication* (2nd edn). Bern: Peter Lang.

Cooter, M. (2000) News notes. *European Science Editions* 26/2, 67.

D'Angelo, L. (2012) Identity conflicts in book reviews: A cross-disciplinary comparison. In M. Gotti (ed.) *Academic Identity Traits: A Corpus-Based Investigation* (pp. 79–94). Bern: Peter Lang.

Eisenberg, D., Davis, R., Ettner, S., Appel, S., Wilkey, S., Rompay, M.V. and Kessler, R. (1998) Trends in alternative medicine use in the United States (1990–1997). *Journal of the American Medical Association* 28/18, 1569–1576.

Ferguson, G., Pérez-Llantada, C. and Plo, R. (2011) English as an international language of scientific publication: A study of attitudes. *World Englishes* 30/1, 41–59.

Fløttum, K. (2006) Medical research articles in the comparative perspectives of discipline and language. In M. Gotti and F. Salager-Meyer (eds) *Advances in Medical Discourse Analysis: Oral and Written Contexts* (pp. 251–269). Bern: Peter Lang.

Giannoni, D. (2008) Medical writing at the periphery: the case of Italian journal editorials. *Journal of English for Academic Purposes* 7/2, 97–107.

Giannoni, D. (2010) Metaphoric values and disciplinary identity in English research articles. In G. Garzone and J. Archibald (eds) *Discourse, Identities and Roles in Specialized Communication* (pp. 281–299). Bern: Peter Lang.

Giannoni, D. (2012) Local/global identities and the medical editorial genre. In M. Gotti (ed.) *Academic Identity Traits: A Corpus-Based Investigation* (pp. 59–78). Bern: Peter Lang.

Goldbeck-Wood, S., Dorozinski, A. and Lie, L.G. (1996) Complementary medicine is booming worldwide. *British Medical Journal* 13, 131–133.

Gotti, M. (2001) The experimental essay in early modern English. *European Journal of English Studies* 5/2, 221–239.

Gotti, M. (2011) *Investigating Specialized Discourse* (3rd edn). Bern: Peter Lang.

Gunnarsson, B.L. (2000) Swedish tomorrow: A product of the linguistic dominance of English? *Current Issues in Language and Society* 7, 51–69.

Hunter, M. (1989) *Establishing the New Science: The Experience of the Early Royal Society.* Woodbridge: Boydell Press.

Hyland, K. (2011) Academic discourse. In K. Hyland and B. Paltridge (eds) *Bloomsbury Companion to Discourse Analysis* (pp. 171–184). London: Continuum.

Jardine, L. (1999) *Ingenious Pursuits: Building the Scientific Revolution.* London: Little, Brown.

Kachru, Y. (2009) Academic writing in world Englishes: The Asian context. In K. Murata and J. Jenkins (eds) *Global Englishes in Asian Contexts* (pp. 111–130). Basingstoke: Palgrave-Macmillan.

Kandiah, T. (2005) Academic writing and global inequality: Resistance, betrayal and responsibility in scholarship. *Language in Society* 34/1, 117–132.

Lefanu, W.R. (1937) British periodicals of medicine: A chronological list. *Bulletin of the Institute of the History of Medicine* 5/8, 735–761 and 5/9, 827–855.

Maci, S.M. (2012) The *discussion* section of medical research articles: A cross-cultural perspective. In M. Gotti (ed.) *Academic Identity Traits: A Corpus-Based Investigation* (pp. 95–120). Bern: Peter Lang.

Mauranen, A. (1993) *Cultural Differences in Academic Rhetoric: A Text Linguistic Study.* Frankfurt am Main: Peter Lang.

Pahta, P. (2006) *This is very important*: A corpus study of amplifiers in medical writing. In M. Gotti and F. Salager-Meyer (eds) *Advances in Medical Discourse Analysis: Oral and Written Contexts* (pp. 357–381). Bern: Peter Lang.

Pérez-Llantada, C. (2012) *Scientific Discourse and the Rhetoric of Globalization: The Impact of Culture and Language.* London: Continuum.

Régent, O. (2000) Pratiques de communication en medicine. *Langages* 105, 66–75.

Rowley-Jolivet, E. and Carter-Thomas, S. (2005) Genre awareness and rhetorical appropriacy: Manipulation of information structure by NS and NNS scientists in the international conference setting. *English for Specific Purposes* 24, 41–64.

Salager-Meyer, F., Alcaraz Ariza, M.Á. and Zambrano, N. (2003) The scimitar, the dagger and the glove: Intercultural differences in the rhetoric of criticism in Spanish, French and English medical discourse (1930–1995). *English for Specific Purposes* 22, 223–247.

Salager-Meyer, F., Alcaraz Ariza, M.A., Pabón, M. and Zambrano, N. (2006) Paying one's intellectual debt: Acknowledgments in scientific/conventional and complementary/alternative medical research. In M. Gotti and F. Salager-Meyer (eds) *Advances in Medical Discourse Analysis: Oral and Written Contexts* (pp. 407–430). Bern: Peter Lang.

Shapiro, B. (2000) *A Culture of Fact: England, 1550–1720.* Ithaca, NY: Cornell University Press.

Swales, J. (1990) *Genre Analysis. English in Academic and Research Settings.* Cambridge: Cambridge University Press.

Swales, J. (1997) English as Tyrannosaurus Rex. *World Englishes* 16, 373–382.

Swales, J. (2004) *Research Genres: Exploration and Applications.* Cambridge: Cambridge University Press.

Taavitsainen, I. and Pahta, P. (eds) (2004) *Medical and Scientific Writing in Late Medieval English.* Cambridge: Cambridge University Press.

Vickers, B. (ed.) (1987) *English Science: Bacon to Newton*. Cambridge: Cambridge University Press.
Vihla, M. (1999) *Medical Writing: Modality in Focus*. Amsterdam: Rodopi.
Webster, C. (1974) *The Intellectual Revolution of the Seventeenth Century*. London: Routledge.
Yakhontova, T. (2001) Textbooks, contexts, and learners. *English for Specific Purposes* 20, 397–415.

3 The Clinical Case Report as a Discourse Genre in the Context of Professional Training[1]

Vicent Salvador

The case study in medical and health settings (clinical case report [CCR]) is a regular section in some specialised academic periodicals. It is a professional genre included as a component in the sequential structure of the macrogenre of 'medical journals', together with editorials, research articles, etc. It is often not rated highly as a scientific contribution because of the epistemological problems raised by processes of non-complete induction; however, it is worthy of interest as a didactic method for improving the skills of students and professionals.

Analysing clinical cases as an actual instance of a therapeutic process is especially relevant in the sphere of studies of communities of practice, a conceptual framework related to the sociology of professional training. From an epistemological and methodological point of view, this conceptual tool is more productive than its relative notion of discourse communities in accounting for the real sociology of health professions. In fact, cooperative groups of colleagues can develop and improve their instructional knowledge (knowing how to do) by means of interactive discourse practices in which exposition, description and narration are the main textual sequences.

My hypothesis highlights the prevalence of the narrative dimension in clinical cases, as a powerful means of making sense of a professional experience and conveying it to readers. The CCR includes the story told by the patient, but it is embedded and elaborated in the framework of the entire discourse to be constructed by a health professional, who selects, interprets and rewords the information provided. The author thereby writes his/her own narrative of the process of sickness and therapy to be read by his/her colleagues. The final statement is usually an evaluation of the results of the treatment.

The study concludes that the CCR, as a medical narrative, contributes to the construction of the patient's identity. From this point of view, the cultivation of the CCR as a genre in medical journals counteracts the tendency towards a mere scientific biomedicine and builds bridges between the two cultures, science and humanities, by establishing a new kind of health study that must have a scientific basis without giving up a personalised conception of the patient as a human subject.

The Clinical Case Report: A Discourse Genre

The genre which is often called the clinical case report (CCR) is a health professional's account of one or more clinical experiences. Morales (2010) provides a brief conceptual approach based on various authors, and a list of the terms most frequently used to designate it: case report, selected report, short report, experience and reason, clinical/scientific note, etc. He also includes the definition given by Khan and Thompson (2002: 849): 'Brief reports describing an isolated clinical case or a small number of cases. They may describe new or uncommon diagnoses, unusual outcomes or prognosis, new or infrequently used therapies and side effects of therapy not usually discovered in clinical trials'.

Both this and other definitions emphasise the novelty or originality of the case described, i.e. its suitability as a relevant contribution to medical science, either because it deals with rare diseases or presents new evidence of symptomatology, etiology or an effective new method of treatment. Jenicek (2001) defines the genre as follows:

> [The CCR] is a form of verbal or written communication with its own specific rules, which is produced for professional and scientific purposes. It usually focuses on an unusual single event (patient or clinical situation) in order to provide a better understanding of the case and of its effects on improved clinical decision-making. (Jenicek, 2001: 93–94)

As we can see, this definition emphasises the newness of the case, but also the aspect of practical application by professionals, while simultaneously signalling the dual possibility that it could be an oral or a written text. In fact, the CCR was both a written and an oral custom for centuries, and played a key role in medical education and communication among professionals. However, the genre, which is today mostly written (although based to a large extent on the patient's oral statements), has been included in the structure of medical journals. In other words, it is published within a composite text in the 'scientific or professional journal' macrogenre (Eggins & Martin, 2003; Salvador *et al.*, 2013) which operates in health settings. CCRs are therefore a piece in a sequence which also contains examples of other genres, such as original research articles, joint reviews, editorials, advertising, etc. Its position in this macro generic framework is not without consequences, as the trend for biomedicine to accept or mimic the parameters of the hard sciences is usually projected onto journals considered elite. As we shall see, in the sphere of the medical journals it is therefore often considered a genre with limited scientific prestige, especially when compared with the research article, which is prototypical of scientific discourse: 'At the extreme "science" end of the genre scale is the research article, the site where new scientific knowledge in medicine is constructed through hypotheses, tested through reliable, usually statistical methods' (Pahta, 2006: 368).

It should also be explained at this point that the concept of genre is understood herein to be a basically actional category, according to a conception that considers language to be a communicative phenomenon linked to (inter-)social activity. Verbal actions take place within social activity, and in addition to being actions in the strictest sense, they can describe other (verbal or non-verbal) actions and resemiotise them. From the perspective of mediated discourse analysis, Scollon (2008: 45) describes it as follows: 'Any discourse analysis, perhaps any analysis of language as it is used, always entails at least some of these relations among human actions and, more importantly, among linguistic descriptions of human actions'. This conception of language – in which the analysis of language is linked to the analysis of social life and vice versa – means that the typology of discourse genres is primarily linked to contexts of action, so that the structural organisation of a text and the stylistic choices of register consistent with the genre will be justified by the configurations typical of these contexts.

Discourse genres understood in these terms are therefore essentially linked to types of actions and contexts, so that their compositional, formal and stylistic characteristics ultimately depend on the actional structure that determines them. This structure has been explicitly or implicitly shaped by the conventions that have configured it over time. The main consequence of this conventionalisation is that the participants in communicative activities related to a particular area of social experience (healthcare environments in this case) automatically recognise the structures of the various genres, and for them they are a preconstruction of discourse. The concept of 'prédiscours' (Paveau, 2006: 118) refers to a set of collective frames (knowledge, beliefs, practices) that are accepted by a community, and which create instructions for producing and interpreting the meaning of discourses. Some of these prior frames coalesce together in each discourse genre, thereby facilitating the identification of this genre as an organic unit by the users of the language, and the genre concerned is often given a commonly accepted designation.

The generic structure of the CCR is very complex. Its origin or primary essence is a chain of events in which prototypically, an interaction occurs between a patient (sometimes with another person who plays the important role of a 'companion') and a healthcare professional. During the first visit, the patient gives a rough description of the origin and the course of the disease that has led him/her to visit the doctor (Salvador & Macián,

2009). The professional, who may have had prior access to some type of clinical documentation (the clinical history, a note written by another healthcare professional who has referred the patient to them, etc.), asks the patient questions during what is called an *anamnesis interview*, takes notes (mentally or physically) of the patient's manifestations, performs a physical examination and perhaps some additional clinical examinations (biochemical analysis, x-rays, etc.) in an attempt to make a diagnosis and determine the most advisable treatment for the disease. Later, in subsequent phases during other clinical encounters, the effectiveness of the treatment applied is observed and some kind of result is produced, which may be positive or negative to a greater or lesser extent. It is therefore an (inter)actional sequence, in which verbal productions (oral or written) alternate with actions of non-verbal communication (eye contact, annotations, gestures, proxemic factors, etc.) and physical examinations (auscultation, palpation, treatments, etc.). This all takes place over a more or less prolonged period of time during successive interactive meetings between the two parties.

To translate this heterogeneous experience into a 'case report', the health professional subsequently performs a complex process of *entextualisation*, which includes procedures such as lexicalisations, nominalisations and various types of resemiotisation (the translation from one system of signs to another) and in short, the construction of a discourse within a framework of communication between specialists. This process profoundly transforms the clinical experience of the professional and the patient, due to a technologisation of the social practice, and the personal identities of those participating.

The CCR originates in the specific oral interactions between the two agents, with questions and answers, which cooperatively generate the illness narrative. However, this narrative subsequently has to be produced by the professional: it thus acquires a different profile when it becomes a written text directed towards one specialist by another, in which the figure of the addresser and the addressee are established, and a different kind of knowledge and new strategies for managing that knowledge among colleagues are created. The discourse thus falls within the sphere of specialisation and of a communication mediated by the genre in medical journals. For example, CCRs describe the 'soft' data obtained from anamnesis and the 'hard' data obtained from laboratory tests. There is often even a 'hardening' of the soft data obtained, when subjective variables such as a pain scale are classified and quantified (Uribarri, 2004).

Biological phenomena thereby become diagnoses, and experiences are structured as a clinical narrative, while the patient becomes a depersonalised and standardised object of study. We could say that patients are 'rewritten' as 'bureaucratic objects', and in extreme cases, their experience of the disease and their personal narrative become electronic medical records: 'It is precisely this aspect of patients' narratives that is sacrificed when they are transformed into the standardized categories of electronic medical records' (Jones, 2013: 139).

Holmes and Ponte (2011) study the training of future medical professionals as regards presentation of the patient, using the process that those authors call 'en-case-ing the patient' –a process in which the patient's words are transferred to a kind of professionalised discourse: 'The transformation of the patient's illness narrative into a biomedical patient presentation can be seen as a ubiquitous instance of medical entextualization' (Holmes & Ponte, 2011: 171). It is the transformation of the illness narrative (and the professional's inferences, evaluations and physical observations regarding the patient) into an academic text aimed at specialists. This manoeuvre requires a prior learning of discursive skills and the effort of *listening* to the patient's body and words at the same time, the selection of data, and interpreting them and giving them a consistency that they often do not have in the original narrative: 'Usually, the story of sickness comes out chaotically, achronologically, and interwoven with bits of life and the past' (Charon, 2006: 99).

Importantly, this is not to say that medical trainees would acquire skills for writing academic texts, but in this way they would learn a major professional skill, i.e. the habit of listening accurately to the patient's casual talk and the capacity to recontextualise his/her narrative in the frame of medical discourse.

The Internal Structure of CCRs

Let us now examine the constituent parts of the textual schema of the prototypical CCR. Pedro Laín Entralgo, a renowned Spanish physician and writer, and a forerunner of today's medical humanities, referred to the structure of what he called the 'pathographical narrative' in a thick volume devoted to the theory and history of the clinical case:

> Hace veinticinco siglos ha sido edificada una estructura de la historia clínica relativamente firme. Repetiré los nombres de sus miembros principales. *Descriptiosubjecti, praegressa remota, origomorbi, praegressaproxima, status praesens, cursusmorbi, exitus*; y cuando éste es letal, añádese a ellos la inspectiocadaveris. (Laín Entralgo, 1998: 738)
>
> [A relatively firm structure of the clinical story has been constructed over the last twenty-five centuries. I will reiterate the names of its main components. *Descriptiosubjecti, praegressaremota, origomorbi, praegressaproxima, status praesens, cursus morbi, exitus*; and when it is lethal, they are joined by the *inspectiocadaveris*]

In Spanish medical literature, Laín Entralgo was responsible for knowledge of an anthropological and humanistic orientation, which argues that the clinical case is a constitutive point in the patient's overall biography. This author adopts a critical attitude towards case reports that are too concise, as he believes that they are similar to aspiring to 'recite Shakespeare in a telegraphic style'. It should be noted that this telegraphic brevity often involves a concealment or misrepresentation of items in the patient's narrative, which may be relevant in various ways: as informative data and as interpretations and assessments of their own pathographic experiences.

After having undergone these changes, the configuration imposed by the genre, as it now appears in specialist journals, corresponds to a kind of text constructed by the doctor, who contextualises the problem within the field of expert knowledge and takes the patient's prior medical history into account. Moreover, the doctor must use the starting point of the patient's narrative of his/her own experience of the problem that he/she brought to the surgery (a narrative that can be elicited by the professional by means of the anamnesis interview). As seen above, this narrative is first recreated by him/her and integrated at a higher enunciative level in their own discourse, in which they interpret the patient's perspective from their own medical perspective, and then include the tests carried out and their own diagnosis and prognosis, and they usually conclude with an attempt to project the results onto a more widespread scenario.

In terms of textual macrostructure, the CCR is a hybrid genre, or at least *textually heterogeneous*, if considered from a theoretical conception of discursive typology, since it usually consists of various types of sequences (Adam, 2011):

(a) *expository* (especially the state of the art and the conclusions with which they often attempt to generalise the knowledge derived from the case study);
(b) *descriptive* (including verbal descriptions and images, usually with a high degree of figurativeness);
(c) finally, the *narrative sequences*, which are particularly relevant and from our point of view can be considered the type of *dominant sequence* in most texts of this genre.

Figure 3.1 shows the prototypical approach in the development of CCRs, where N_0 represents the patient's narrative, an illness narrative, while N_1 is the medical narrative that incorporates and recontextualises it.

According to this theory, the narrative is the dominant sequence in texts in this genre, the most specific characteristic of the case report and is therefore a member of the family of narrative discourses, and the subject of a powerful modern paradigm in the study of academic and professional discourses, including medical discourse (Gotti & Sancho Guinda, 2013). The importance of narrative for communication in health settings has often been emphasised, for example in relation to the narratives of the chronically ill (Lonardi, 2006) and also with respect to CCRs, which are

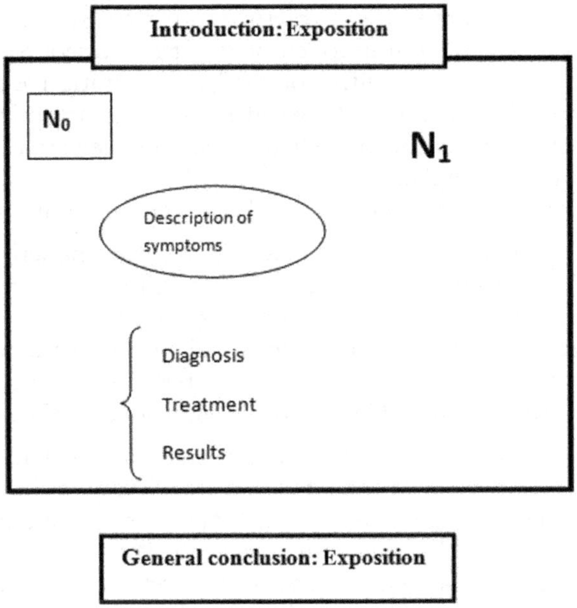

Figure 3.1 Diagram of the prototypical internal structure of a CCR

considered a narrative genre which transforms one narrative into another one that is more abstract and professionalised:

> This particular narrative genre consists of a story that begins with a succession of events or experiences relating to the patient, which then becomes progressively abstracted from the patient's control and the context of its original telling. The extracted story progresses,transformed by a medicotechnical vocabulary not likely to be understood by the patient. (Hurwitz, 2000: 2088)

As discussed below, the inclusion of the study of this genre in narrative-focused studies leads us to consider the specificity and validity of narrative as a way of thinking about reality, in comparison with the logical, scientific way of constructing discourse and its world view. Academic training and the essential practical training of health professionals must combine both discursive and cognitive styles productively and efficiently.

Returning to the approach in Figure 3.1, the professional weaves together the narrative story of the patient's anamnesis, the treatment and its outcome (N_1), selecting the data and presenting the facts in a systematic and coherent way, using the chronological sequence as a basic schema and establishing causal relationships between the events (as much as possible, and often hypothetically). The language used is that of the specialist, and the time coordinates are those of the time in which the report is written. The materials that they use to construct their discourse include the narrative of the patient, who either on his/her own initiative or in response to questions by the professional, provides the necessary information and generally concludes with the immediate reason for the patient's visit to the doctor, or the chief complaint.

The mechanism of this enunciative inclusion can be summarised as follows:

Narrative$_0$: Clinical history referred by the patient or possible companion (and often supplemented with a clinical history from other professionals). Critical point: the reason for the visit.

Narrative$_1$: Narrative of the professional, covering the entire process (clinical history, chief complaint, clinical tests, diagnosis, progress of treatment and final results). **Narrative$_0$** is embedded in **Narrative$_1$**.

The illness narrative (N_0) is thereby *recontextualised* in the medical narrative by a selection of the elements that are relevant in the professional's opinion, a coherent arrangement of the facts and an evaluative interpretation. The patient's voice is therefore subsumed into that of the doctor. Then, the patient's sentences are narrated as facts or reported indirectly, as in the following text taken from Hurwitz (2000), who uses it as a brief example of a clinical tale:

> A 75-year-old man **told** me he was being kept awake by the sound of machinery emanating from the right side of his chest. He could hear the noise only at night. It was not accompanied by any other sensation and, clinically, it was inaudible to me. (Hurwitz, 2000: 2086)

Here, the doctor reports the patient's words in indirect speech, introduced by the locative verb 'told', in a very neutral manner. Interestingly, the information is relevant, particularly because of the doctor's description of the patient's pectoral noise –'clinically, it was inaudible to me'.

In some texts, the locative verb is not as neutral as in the example above, and may include semantic paradigms such as 'to admit', 'to confess' and 'to deny'. The latter verb is used in the example below, where the fact that the patient denies smoking and alcoholism is presented as a testimony for which the patient is solely responsible, while the reporter does not necessarily appear to accept the veracity of the statement:

> Hombre de 73 años de edad, chofer federal, tabaquismo y alcoholismo **negados**. Hipertenso de 20 años de evolución en tratamiento con telmisartán y ácido acetilsalicílico. Jugador de fútbol hasta los 68 años de edad. Se le realizó coronariografa en 1999 en México, D. F. sin encontrar lesiones coronarias. A los 53 años de edad presentó palpitaciones de inicio súbito, rápidas, posterior a jugar partido de fútbol que requirió de

> tratamiento médico para revertir la taquicardia. Posteriormente presentó tres eventos más hasta marzo de 2008, que ameritó hospitalización y tratamiento IV en el Hospital ISSSTE de Puebla, con lo cual revirtió a ritmo sinusal. (Reyes *et al.*, 2009: 92)
>
> [A 73-year-old man, a driver for the federal government, **denied** smoking and alcoholism. Hypertensive for more than 20 years in treatment with telmisartan and acetylsalicylic acid. Played football until 68 years old. He underwent coronary angiography in Mexico City in 1999, with no coronary lesions observed. At 53 years old he presented sudden fast palpitations after playing a football match, which required medical treatment to reverse the tachycardia. He subsequently presented three more events until March 2008, which required hospitalization and IV therapy in the ISSSTE Hospital in Puebla, after which sinus rhythm was restored.]

In other cases, the locative verb which supposedly introduces the statements of N_0 has been erased, and what is presented is a mere statement of the facts, albeit one that is obviously based on the patient's testimony, as in the following example:

> A 54-year-old asymptomatic man with a 5-year history of type 2 diabetes mellitus (T2DM) was found to have an extremely low serum cholesterol concentration. He had no history of major childhood illness, malabsorption, or any cardiovascular or neurologic dysfunction. He had smoked for 30 years and was not using alcohol or any lipid-lowering drugs. Additionally, he was not a vegetarian. His family history included stroke (father died at age 52 years) and chronic kidney disease (57-year-old brother). His eldest son had died of a suspected myocardial infarction at the age of 21 years. (Turk *et al.*, 2012: 826)

In some instances, the report presents the evolution of a disease over many years and various episodes, in a summary focusing on that particular aspect of the person's health, together with the results of the process and sometimes interspersed with an explicit locative verb ('reported') which is elided elsewhere ('also'), thereby activating the assumption that the facts narrated by the author of the report (N_1) are known due to a previous narrative (N_0):

> In the 1980s, a woman in her 40s started noticing that her hats were not fitting. She ***also* reported** suffering from headache, hearing loss and tinnitus. Alkaline phosphatase and urinary hydroxyproline levels were raised in the beginning. She was diagnosed with Paget's disease. [...] After three decades, the skull bones grew as seen in figures 1 and 2. [...] Currently, there are no signs of activity of the disease. (Maia *et al.*, 2014: 1)

A very important point in the clinical case occurs when the professional's narrative mentions the patient's chief complaint leading him/her to seek medical help ('he/she attended the unit ... due to...').

Generally, the relevant transition point where the reference of N_1 to N_0 is no longer perceived occurs at the point at which a reference to physical examinations, clinical trials and their evaluation begins, as in the following text. At this point in the narrative, the echo of the patient's voice is lost, and the physician's voice becomes the only one that is heard:

> Anamnesis: varón de 51 años de edad previamente sano y sin antecedentes personales ni familiares, únicamente admite haber bebido agua de una acequia una semana antes. Desde entonces está con dolor abdominal y deposiciones diarreicas. Últimamente ha comenzado con vómitos y fiebre. *Exploración física*: buen estado general... (Martínez Cañamero *et al.*, 2011: 190)

> [Anamnesis: a 51-year-old previously healthy male with no personal or family history, who only admits to having drunk water from a ditch a week earlier. He has suffered from abdominal pain and loose stools since then. He has recently begun to experience vomiting and fever. **Physical examination:** good general health...]

The account of events is sometimes complicated because there is more than one source of information and voice in N_0, such as in cases when one of these sources is the companion, as occurs in the following text, with the testimony of the patient's husband and the prior medical history, which includes references to factors of social biographical history:

> A middle aged geriatric male person reported to the department of prosthodontics seeking a solution for his spouse. The female patient, aged 64 years old, living presently with her husband, was suffering from dementia without undergoing any medical treatment, was completely edentulous since last 7 years (Figure 1). Medical history was non-contributory to dental treatment, though the severity of dementia was significant as revealed by her spouse. Social history revealed that the couples were staying alone as their children were settled in other respective places. Due to economic reasons, the spouse of the patient was not available at home during the day time. Examination revealed that the patient had lost her teeth earlier than anticipated due to oral neglect. The patient had been wearing dentures in the past but with passage of time and onset of dementia, was unable to use them efficiently due to which she had lost considerable weight since last 6 months. Significant findings in the history included forgetting to cook, eat or drink, forgetting self-care needs like hygiene maintenance, nutrient, diet

> intake and many other day to day activities. Two areas of concern for her spouse were that the patient would forget the actual wearing of dentures as well as their use. After thorough diagnosis, treatment plan included incorporation of a visual identifier in the complete denture prosthesis that the patient would wear in the form of prefabricated occlusal surfaces. (Mattoo *et al.*, 2014: 194–195)

The complexity of the narrative, even if it consists of a text coming from a single speaker, may be due to the report including the patient's own observations in detail, his/her subjective assessment of the experience. In some cases, the text may include a literal phrase that reveals the exact form of the words of N_0. By all means, this consideration of the patient's expression and opinions is intensified when it is a very serious disease that calls his/her identity into question (e.g. some types of cancer) or when psychosomatic or neurological factors come into play, as in the example below which refers to the feeling of 'déjà vu' experienced by the patient:

> We present the case of a 23-year-old White British man who presented with persistent déjà vu in 2010. He reported experiencing these symptoms since early 2007 shortly after starting university. He had a history of feeling anxious, particularly in relation to contamination, which led him to wash his hands very frequently and to shower two to three times per day, and his anxiety worsened around the time he began university. Anxiety and low mood led him to take a break from university, and he then began experiencing déjà vu. His recollection of these early episodes was that they would last for minutes, but could also be extremely prolonged. For example, while on holiday in a destination that he had previously visited he reported feeling as though he had become 'trapped in a time loop'. He reported finding these experiences very frightening.
>
> He returned to university in 2007 and he described the déjà vu episodes as becoming more intense. He took lysergic acid diethylamide (LSD) once, and from then on the déjà vu was fairly continuous.
>
> [.......]
>
> He was assessed by AZ in 2010, at which point his persistent déjà vu caused him to avoid watching television and listening to the radio, as well as reading papers and magazines, as he felt he had already encountered the content before. His neurological examination was normal. At the time of assessment he reported a chronically low mood and felt anxious much of the time, although his compulsive behaviours were not a problem. There was a family history of obsessive compulsive disorder (OCD) on his paternal and possibly maternal side. (Wells *et al.*, 2014: 2–3)

Another example, which also presents psychological aspects and finally had no satisfactory resolution, shows us how the inclusion and absorption of the patient's discourse can lead to a vast, complex text that is full of appreciative nuances. The subject of the CCR is an adolescent teenager ('C.A.') afflicted with an obsessive-compulsive disorder (OCD), that is, an anxiety disorder that involves (a) intrusive unwanted thoughts, ideas or images that evoke anxiety (obsessions); and (b) deliberate behavioural or mental rituals to neutralise this distress (compulsion). After presenting the theoretical framework of this ailment, the authors of the text discuss the patient's chief complaints, and reproduce his words synthetically using indirect speech:

> C.A. stated that he was constantly bothered by thoughts of suffering brain damage and participating in immoral acts. In addition, he was spending a great deal of time trying to avoid activities that might suggest that he had brain damage and to minimize the chances that he would get brain damage. Although C.A. had been a good student who enjoyed learning, he was currently having difficulty in school because of his OCD symptoms. He also reported no longer reading for enjoyment, which was one of his favourite activities. (Whiteside & Abramowitz, 2006: 525)

The text then reviews the young man's family history (upper-middle-class, small town in the Midwestern US, Christian community, an older brother, etc.). It notes that his mother described him as 'somewhat shy and introverted' and adds other details from the patient's statements and the observation conducted by the therapist:

> He appeared to have a supportive family and denied any history of abuse or trauma. There was no evidence that C.A. was using alcohol or illegal drugs. C.A. recalled that his OCD symptoms began in the first grade, when he experienced persistent concerns about germs that led to frequent hand washing. (Whiteside & Abramowitz, 2006: 525)

In the section entitled 'Assessment', the authors combine theoretical and methodological considerations using the academic discourse of the genre and references to the patient's responses to questions asked by the therapist, in an attempt to elicit information that could help to fill the gaps in the adolescent's spontaneous narrative and interpret them correctly:

> It is also important to evaluate the patient fear-based avoidance and appraisal of his or her intrusive thoughts when developing a case formulation. [...] First, the therapist inquired about external cues

> that triggered C.A.'s intrusive thoughts. C.A. reported that cleaning solutions, lead paint, insect repellent, and other household solvents and objects provoked obsessional thoughts about brain damage. [...] In addition, C.A. reported that when in the company of his family, he had unwanted thoughts of engaging in sexual intercourse. Finally, information about drugs evoked unwanted doubts that perhaps he had used street drugs in the past or would do so in the future, which he felt was immoral and might lead to brain damage. (Whiteside & Abramowitz, 2006: 526)

Elsewhere in the presentation of the case, the authors directly and literally reproduce a sequence of 'Socratic questioning' by the patient's therapist (one of the two authors of the article):

> **S.W. (author):** What about these thoughts makes you nervous?
> **C.A.:** It would be bad to do drugs or have brain damage.
> **S.W.:** Yes, it would, but is talking about it or thinking about it the same as doing drugs or having brain damage?
> **C.A.:** No, I guess not. (Whiteside & Abramowitz, 2006: 532)

Obviously, the more heavily that psychological issues are involved in the clinical case and the less that strictly biomedical issues are involved, the greater the need for accuracy and precision when reproducing the patient's narrative. However, the boundary between the two types of case is undoubtedly vague, at least from a holistic conception of the individual and an overall assessment of the expression of the patient's identity.

However, the most striking conclusion from an examination of the various samples analysed is that the enunciative density of the text of the CCR is apparent, and that the professional's wording has to recontextualise the various voices that it includes and resemiotise the non-verbal elements of the discourse, which is essentially narrative. The sequence of events and the causal relationships established between them thus make a mosaic of pieces into a coherent and interpreted evaluative whole, so that its publication leads to a contribution to medical knowledge. That will be more evident if the case narrated has a happy therapeutic ending, and if this is the case, the status of the health professional communicating the experience to colleagues will obviously be reinforced. More successful cases than failed ones are undoubtedly published, but we should not forget that failures or incomplete successes, like the last one discussed above, highlight errors and thus contain very useful practical lessons, as we shall see below:

> Publishing an unsuccessful case description is more difficult than publishing a successful one. Successful case descriptions are usually

> modelled on the theories on which the prescription was based. Successful cases may be more comforting, but unsuccessful cases are indispensable for estimating the reliability of our prescribing indications, and their practical usefulness. (Baas, 2004: 25)

The Role of the CCR in Professional Training

As hinted at above, the CCR as a genre does not enjoy high prestige among media purely focusing on research. This is because it is a 'case study' (an analysis of a single case or a very small selection of cases) and, as it occurs in other disciplines, it can hardly justify the drawing of conclusions of a general nature, insofar as it corresponds to a process of *incomplete induction* (which is, in fact, very incomplete).

In the dialectic between qualitative and quantitative methods, the procedure is positioned squarely on the side of the former (Niero, 2008). This indicates that the genre does not conform to the dominant trends in the world of biomedicine, which is today more prone to quantification and statistics. However, its dual quality of research and dissemination (or as a teaching method for professional training) also reduces its prestige in fields considered scientific, such as in specialised journals, which at most include texts about special cases that are very rarely covered in the literature, but do not include contributions about subjects that are generally applicable. In their editorial, some medical journals insist on the need for CCRs to have a high degree of originality in their content if they are to be published, as stated in this editorial:

> Creo que los autores, antes de mandar un caso clínico, deberían analizar si es absolutamente novedoso, es decir, si algunos de sus aspectos (diagnósticos, terapéuticos) no han sido previamente publicados. Es habitual que ante un caso clínico raro tengamos la sensación de haber descubierto algo muy importante, que generosamente queremos compartir con los colegas en forma de publicación. Sin embargo, muchas veces, cuando revisamos profundamente la bibliografía previa (que es, por cierto, muy abundante), casi siempre llegamos a la conclusión de que algún caso similar (o varios) ya han sido publicados y que en realidad el nuestro aporta poco o nada a los lectores con respecto a lo ya conocido. (Rodríguez-Merchán, 2005: 241)
>
> [I believe that before sending a clinical case, the authors should consider whether it is absolutely new, i.e. whether some aspects (diagnostic and therapeutic) have not been previously published. It is common when dealing with a rare clinical case to have the feeling of having discovered something very important that we generously want to share with colleagues in the form of a publication. However, when

> we carry out an in-depth review of the literature (which is indeed very abundant), we almost always reach the conclusion that a similar case (or several) has already been published, and in fact ours contributes little or nothing to readers in terms of what they already know.]

This requirement for newness, which is reasonable from the point of view of the progress of scientific knowledge in the strict sense, is contradictory to the educational value of 'classic' clinical cases as an example provided in classrooms with the aim to establish a theory or a protocol for diagnosis and treatment in the minds of students of medicine or other health sciences. They are illustrations that are fixed in the learners' memory, as used in the manuals covering various disciplines. Indeed, CCRs are often illustrations of theory and application exercises in university lecture rooms or trivial contributions to professional retraining. One of the reasons behind the prejudice towards the influx of CCRs as candidates for publication among journals with claims to scientificity is that they are often the first works produced by a novice researcher who is not yet confident enough to write original research articles.

It has even often been noted that the eminently narrative nature of the CCR makes it less argumentative and less critical than other genres in the specialist journal macrogenre, thus making it the most uncritical genre because it incorporates the least amount of negative appraisals. However, Piqué-Angordans and Posteguillo (2006) found some critical examples in their corpus that are largely self-critical statements, which would suggest that the genre can be described as a discourse that is less pretentious and more cautious in its conclusions:

> However, these instantiations of negative evaluative comments are not all addressed to other fellow researchers, but most of them are used as a means to express self-criticism. This self-critical approach may be conveyed on a direct personal style, with expressions like 'although questionable, our plan was' and 'our lack of experience'. (Piqué-Angordans & Posteguillo, 2006: 393–394)

Nevertheless, despite the humility of a genre that is considered minor in some scientific fields, in professional journals (which are to some extent the continuation of specialised teaching, a kind of lifelong learning or retraining during the professional career), their appeal is interesting for several reasons, as has been studied with regard to chiropody (Macián, 2015). First, because the aims of these publications include fostering the group cohesion of the profession, and to do so it is important to disseminate practical knowledge, and second, because of the ease of access for its readers/subscribers to the publication of their own work. As a result, what would be a fault from a strictly scientific perspective becomes an advantage within the discursive construction of the professional cohesion, if considered from the perspective of a sociology of the professions (Champy, 2011; Rodriguez, 2008).

Indeed, it has been empirically confirmed that in some journals of this type, such as *Atención Primaria*, aimed at professionals working in general medicine, the most widely read articles are in fact those in this genre (Salvador *et al.*, 2013). Furthermore, online journals dedicated specifically to the publication of this kind of discourse have appeared in recent years, such as *BMJ Case Reports*, *American Journal of Case Reports* and *Journal of Medical Case Reports*, from which we extracted some examples for our analysis. All of these factors contribute to an improved definition of the specific characteristics of professional discourse in comparison to scientific or academic discourse (Gunnarsson, 2009; López Ferrero, 2002; Parodi, 2010).

The current boom in the genre studied here should be understood in the social context of what is known as communities of practice (Martos, 2012; Wenger, 1998), which is a more specific concept than discourse communities (Swales, 1990), as it involves cooperation between peers and is focused more on 'knowing how to do' than on theoretical knowledge. Professional journals are an appropriate forum for the exchange of problem-solving experiences, which are not limited to illustrating theories but also present the procedures by which medical colleagues have attempted to establish diagnoses and apply therapies, with a value as a practical example that is considerable in other situations comparable to those presented in a specific case. Learning thus becomes a procedural learning based on personal testimony: the clinician's, who when reporting the facts includes his/her own path of discovery and of questioning of the possible interpretations that enable an account of the case to be given, and of its compliance with a model of scientific explanation that is satisfactory.

In this respect, the CCR has a characteristic virtue that other types of medical discourse do not have: it presents *in vivo* a discovery process, where what is important is not so much the results (more or less successful) of a diagnosis and therapeutic treatment. It is also possible to learn from failures, if the researcher makes the methodology followed clear. What good CCRs teach is how to conduct a practical research procedure, which uses raw data, and in which the patient's testimony is very important in order to construct a coherent interpretation in an attempt to solve a problem. An editorial explains it as follows:

> Para el clínico experimentado, el reto está en reconocer lo sutil, el paciente no tan clásico, con una actitud semejante al arquetipo *Sherlock Holmes* para resolver un caso desconcertante. [...] La realidad es que muchos *casos clásicos* no se reconocen inicialmente, sino que son

> identificados como tales después de que se ha ensamblado las piezas de la evidencia diagnóstica. Este es un proceso que inevitablemente se despliega en el tiempo, con muchos giros y vueltas, tentaciones que nos llevan a caminos con callejones sin salida frustrantes. En los ejercicios de la enseñanza formal, la historia clínica es presentada en forma total, dando a los estudiantes una perspectiva global después de compilar todo el proceso diagnóstico. Casos como este carecen del desarrollo cronológico del proceso de enfermedad, lo simplifican en exceso y distorsionan la realidad del aprendizaje y la práctica del diagnóstico clínico. Es precisamente la capacidad para reconstruir la dimensión del tiempo lo que permite, al menos en parte, agregar un valor educativo a lo que se ha denominado ejercicios de resolución de problemas clínicos introducido por el Dr. Jerome Kassirer y sus colegas en la prestigiosa revista *The New England Journal of Medicine* hace varios años. (Bosques Padilla, 2010: 89–90)
>
> [For the experienced clinician, the challenge lies in recognizing the subtle case, the patient who is not a classic case, using an attitude similar to the archetype of *Sherlock Holmes* when solving a baffling case. [...] The fact is that many *classic cases* are not initially recognized, but are instead identified as such after the pieces of diagnostic evidence have been assembled. This is a process that inevitably takes time, with many twists and turns, and temptations that lead to frustrating dead ends. In formal teaching exercises, the clinical history is presented in its entirety, giving students an overall perspective, after compiling the entire diagnostic process. Cases like this one lack the chronological development of the disease's evolution, they oversimplify it and distort real learning conditions and clinical diagnosis. It is precisely the ability to reconstruct the dimension of time that at least partially enables an educational value to be added to what have been called exercises in clinical problem-solving, introduced by Dr. Jerome Kassirer and his colleagues in the prestigious journal *The New England Journal of Medicine* several years ago.]

This leads us back to the thesis of this chapter: the predominantly narrative nature of CCRs, as other scholars have pointed out (Goyal, 2013). It is a narrative of a specific process of inquiry, based on the patient's narrative, defined and recontextualised by the author and continued by the narrative of the subsequent diagnostic and therapeutic process. Telling a story (in which another one is embedded) is a way – another way – of discovering reality. As Gabriel (2013) reminds us, a community of practitioners is also a community of storytellers or story researchers.

This reflection enables us to rise to a more abstract level of discussion: the epistemological value of narrative as a model for discourse, compared to the logical, explanatory value of the science with which it undoubtedly complements the venturing of knowledge. The narrative model is idiographic rather than nomothetic, and does not easily allow the mechanism of Popperian falsification. It is more similar to the jurisprudence established by the courts of law than to positive laws, and it makes a different type of contribution to knowledge. Its great virtue is that – to use Dilthey's terminology – it is oriented towards *understanding* rather than towards providing an *explanation* by means of observable generalisations. The backdrop is the long theoretical and methodological debate between the 'two cultures' of science and the humanities, which also takes place in the social sciences: 'These different approaches – a hermeneutic-reconstructive one on the one hand (understanding) and a nomothetic-deductive one on the other hand (explaining) – have practically drawn a dividing line through the modern social sciences' (Weiss & Wodak, 2003: 2). The sphere of understanding necessarily contains ample room for interpretation.

Narrative, Identities and Literature

In the preceding sections, we have seen the extent to which the concept of narrative is inseparable from the CCR, and more broadly, from a conception of medical practice in which narrative skills have a decisive influence. Indeed, the term 'narrative medicine' has recently gained currency and has been succinctly defined by Rita Charon (2006: 4) as follows: 'I use the term *narrative medicine to* mean medicine practised with these narrative skills of recognizing, absorbing, interpreting, and being moved by the stories of illness'. Indeed, narrative captures the singular and the irreplicable items in human life and thus plays a role of nourishing knowledge that is different from generalisations about science.

When the CCR falls within this conception of medicine, it reflects or reconstructs a pathographical narrative that is a part of the patient's overall (auto)biography – a piece of their personal identity. As we have seen, it does so by including it within the narrative of a broader process, in which the patient's individual experience should not be neglected in favour of medical nomenclature and the pursuit of the scientific approach. If the doctor is able to listen to the patient, their ability to solve the problem of their disease will increase decisively.

Jerome Groopman's book (2007) entitled *How Doctors Think*, which focuses on the issue of physician–patient communication as a prerequisite for good medical practice, has recently achieved an extraordinarily high level of circulation and impact. The author argues that the physician's practical knowledge must combine science and experience with good communication with the patient, the ability to patiently question the patient and listen carefully to avoid diagnostic errors: 'doctoring is an art'. The book develops this idea and establishes an effective and ethical perspective for the profession, which is primarily intended for laypeople but undoubtedly useful for health professionals.

In the first pages of his book, Groopman (2007: 2) tells the story of a patient who was diagnosed 'with anorexia nervosa with bulimia' and went from doctor to doctor for 15 years: 'Anne was also evaluated by numerous specialists: endocrinologists, orthopaedists, haematologists, infectious disease doctors, and, of course, psychologists and psychiatrists. [...] But Anne's health continued to deteriorate, and the past twelve months had been the most miserable of her life'. After continuing the ordeal with a progressive deterioration of her health, she was saved by her meeting with Dr Falchuk. The gastroenterologist ignored the instructions of the specialist who had referred the patient to him, and instead of continuing the chain due to the momentum of inertia, began to prepare a new diagnosis from the beginning, listening carefully and dialogically to the patient's narrative: 'But that is exactly what Falchuk did not do. Instead, he began to question, and listen, and observe, and then to think differently about Anne's case. And by doing so, he saved her life, because for fifteen years a key aspect of her illness had been missed' (Groopman, 2007: 3). The narratives of this type that Groopman includes in his book act to some extent as an *exempla* that provide a lesson in behaviour. They are narratives based on clinical cases, but which are written with an expressive force, i.e. to a certain extent made literary, which is why they are more accessible to the public at large.

This is a similar strategy to the one used in several books by the neurologist Oliver Sacks, whose work has gained widespread circulation, without its author's reputation as a researcher being compromised. This work aims to radically change the current perspective of neurology and medicine in general, and raise awareness of the need to consider the patient's subjectivity and identity. This attitude reflects a change in the demands of today's society: 'A significant innovation in medical practice has been the movement for "patient-centred" medicine which aims to give more room for the voicing of patient concerns and perspectives in the medical encounter' (Heritage & Clayman, 2010: 155).

Sacks (1985) develops a humanist vision of the relationship with the patient, using narratives that are located between the clinical case and the story, making use of a wide variety of resources found in literary rhetoric, ranging from striking metaphorisation to intrigue, to almost surreal titles (Salvador, in press). An example of this technique can be seen in this excerpt from his most famous work, *The Man Who Mistook His Wife for a Hat*, and specifically at the start of one of the narratives consisting of a patient's clinical history before coming to the surgery:

> Bhagawhandi P, an Indian girl of 19 with a malignant brain tumour, was admitted to our hospice in 1978. The tumour –an astrocytoma– had first presented when she was seven, but was then of low malignancy, and well circumscribed, allowing a complete resection, and complete return of function, and allowing Bhagawhandi to return to normal life.
>
> This reprieve lasted for ten years, during which she lived life to the full, lived it gratefully and consciously to the full, for she knew (she was a bright girl) that she had a 'time bomb' in her head,
>
> In her eighteenth year, the tumour recurred, much more invasive and malignant now, and no longer removable. A decompression was performed to allow its expansion –and it was with this, with weakness and numbness of the left side, with occasional seizures and other problems that Bhagawhandi was admitted. (Sacks, 1985: 146)

The clinical history is narrated here concisely and at the same time with the fluency of the novelist, and does not hesitate to use expressive metaphors like 'a time-bomb in her head'. An extract of the narrative that begins the aforementioned book and gives it its title follows. This is the point at which the patient-protagonist is referred to the neurologist-narrator, who conveys to the readers the impression created by the symptoms observed in the patient during their first meeting:

> It was obvious within a few seconds of meeting him that there was no trace of dementia in the ordinary sense. He was a man of great cultivation and charm, who talked well and fluently, with imagination and humour. I couldn't think why he had been referred to our clinic.
>
> And yet there *was* something a bit odd. He faced me as he spoke, was oriented toward me, and yet there was something the matter –it was difficult to formulate. He faced me with his *ears*, I came to think, but not with his eyes. These, instead of looking, gazing, at me,, 'taking me in, in the normal way, made sudden strange fixation –on my nose, on my right ear, down to my chin, up to my right eye– as if noting (even studying) these individual features, but not seeing my whole face, its changing expressions, 'me' as a whole. I am not sure that I fully realized this at the time –there was just a teasing strangeness, some failure in the normal interplay of gaze and expression. He saw me, he scanned me, and yet... (Sacks, 1985: 8)

Immediately afterwards, the narrator-neurologist asks about the chief complaint which has led the patient to come to the surgery. This is a key moment in the presentation of the case, but the patient appears to be disoriented and does not know how to respond. The neurologist, who momentarily leaves the room to consult the patient's companion, then describes the patient's contemplative reaction and tells us, before the physical examination, about the delightful impression his attitude makes on him:

> 'What seems to be the matter?' I asked him at length.
>
> 'Nothing that I know of', he replied with a smile, 'but people seem to think that there's something wrong with my eyes.'
>
> 'But *you* don't recognise any visual problems?'
>
> 'No, not directly, but I occasionally make mistake.'
>
> I left the room briefly, to talk to his wife. When I came back Dr P. was sitting placidly by the window, attentive, listening rather than looking out. 'Traffic', he said, 'street sounds, distant trains – they make a sort of symphony, do they not? You know Honegger's Pacific 234?'
>
> What a lovely man, I thought to myself. How can there be anything seriously the matter? Would he permit me to examine him?
>
> Yes, of course, Dr Sacks.' (Sacks, 1985: 8)

Using these procedures, taken from his own professional experience and the resources that literary narrative provides, it is as if Sacks seduces the reader while engaging in pedagogy, becoming a disseminator of a new attitude to the practice of medicine – and of the CCR in particular – as a commitment to a new medical humanism that caters to personal identity: 'We have, each of us, a life-story, an inner narrative – whose continuity, whose sense, *is* our lives. It may be said that each of us constructs and lives, a "narrative", and that this narrative is our identities' (Sacks, 1985: 105).

Conclusion

After all these considerations, it can be stated that the CCR – providing that it is not a telegraphic document – contributes to the patient's *pathography*, is a variant of the biography and for that reason contributes to the construction of his/her identity (as a patient and as a person). Its function, like that of many other narratives, is to understand the patient by interpreting data and the episodes of his/her pathography.

If we think of medicine as a discipline that is more concerned with the illness of each patient than with diseases understood in terms of theoretical objects of study, doctors cannot refuse to personalise their professional practice, or the exercise of prudence (the classical concept of *phronesis*, one of the three branches of knowledge described by Aristotle) that the profession requires. Indeed, as well as *episteme* and *techne*, *phronesis* is the opposite of acting mechanically based on scripts and protocols, and is a specifically human factor that completes medical practice:

> If *episteme* is of the head, *techne* is of the hand. *Techne* invokes making; it produces objects, originally art-works and what we now call technology. Surgery, as a craftwork of the hands, is a form of *techne*. *Techne* teaches how to craft, and *episteme* teaches the laws that govern what is crafted, but neither form of knowledge takes us very far in deciding what we ought to craft. For that we need *phronesis*. (Frank, 2004: 221)

For Victoria Camps (2007), this concept of *phronesis* is one of the essential virtues of the medical professions – a virtue that enables it to address the complexity of healing, beyond the knowledge of an expert in an applied science, and which helps to build a professional *ethos* that is ethically and socially committed. From this perspective, the cultivation of the CCR as a genre counteracts the tendency towards a 'veterinary' medicine and builds bridges between the two cultures, science and humanities, by establishing new kinds of health studies that must undoubtedly have a scientific basis, but without giving up a personalised conception of the patient as a subject and an unavoidable ethical commitment to society.

Note

(1) Research project 'Retórica constructivista: discursos de la identidad'(FFI 2013-40934-R). Research project 'Lenguaje y cultura de la salud' (CSO2014-61928-EXP).

References

Adam, J.M. (2011) *Les textes: types et prototypes*. Paris: Armand Colin.

Baas, V. (2004) The pitfalls of clinical case research: Lessons from the Delphi Project. *Homeopathy* 93, 21–25.

Bosques Padilla, F.J. (2010) Resolución de casos clínicos como una estrategia para la enseñanza de la medicina. *Medicina Universitaria* 12 (47), 89–90.

Camps, V. (2007) La excelencia en las profesiones sanitarias. *Humanitas. Humanidades Médicas* 21, 1–13.

Champy, F. (2011) *Nouvelle théorie sociologique des professions*. Paris: Presses Universitaires de France.

Charon, R. (2006) *Narrative Medicine. Honoring the Stories of Illness*. Oxford: Oxford University Press.

Eggins, S. and Martin, J.R. (2003) El contexto como género. Una propuesta de lingüística funcional. *Revista Signos* 35 (54), 185–205.

Frank, A.W. (2004) Asking the right question about pain: Narrative and phronesis. *Literature and Medicine* 23 (2), 209–225.

Gabriel, Y. (2013) Storytelling in organizational research. In M. Gotti and C. Sancho Guinda (eds) *Narratives in Academic and Professional Genres* (pp. 105–122). Bern: Peter Lang.

Gotti, M. and Sancho Guinda, C. (eds) (2013) *Narratives in Academic and Professional Genres*. Bern: Peter Lang.

Goyal, R. (2013) Narration in medicine. In P. Hühn, J. Pier, W. Schmid and J. Schönert (eds) *The Living Handbook of Narratology*. Hamburg: Hamburg University.

Groopman, J. (2007) *How Doctors Think*. Boston, MA: Houghton Mifflin.

Gunnarsson, B.L. (2009) *Professional Discourse*. London: Continuum.

Heritage, J. and Clayman, S. (2010) *Talk in Action. Interactions, Identities, and Institutions*. Oxford: Wiley-Blackwell.

Holmes, S.M. and Ponte, M. (2011) En-case-ing the patient: Disciplining uncertainty in medical student patient presentations. *Cult Med Psyquiatry* 35, 163–182.

Hurwitz, B. (2000) Narrative and the practice of medicine. *Lancet* 356, 2086–2089.

Jenicek, M. (2001) *Clinical Case Reporting in Evidence-Based Medicine* (2nd edn). London: Arnold.

Jones, R.H. (2013) *Health and Risk Communication. An Applied Linguistic Perspective*. New York: Routledge.

Khan, K. and Thompson, P. (2002) A proposal for writing and appraising case reports. *British Journal of Obstetrics and Gynaecology* 109, 849–851.

Laín Entralgo, P.(1998) *La historia clínica. Historia y teoría del relato patográfico*, Madrid: Triacastela (original work published 1950).

Lonardi, C. (2006) *Racconti di cefalea. Approchio bibliografico alla malattia cronica*. Verona: QuiEdit.

López Ferrero, C. (2002) Aproximación al análisis de los discursos profesionales. *Revista Signos* 35 (51–52), 195–215.

Macián, C. (2015) La construcción discursiva de la profesión podológica: aplicación al análisis de un corpus de revistas especializadas. PhD Universitat Jaume I. See http://www.tdx.cat/handle/10803/285099 (accessed 14 March 2015).

Maia, J.M., Alves, R., Faria, R. and Farinha, F. (2014) She could no longer wear a hat: Paget's disease. *BMJ Case Reports*, doi:10.1136/bcr-2014-207515, 1–2. See http://www.ncbi.nlm.nih.gov/pubmed/25410038 (accessed 30 April 2015).

Martínez Cañamero, A., Gasso Campos, M., Aguilar Peña, R., Herrera Contreras, I., Moral Eliche, A., Camacho Reina, M.V. and Peña Casas, A.M. (2011) Síndrome de respuesta inflamatoria sistémica en adulto sano. *Revista del Laboratorio Clínico (Especial Congreso) Comunicaciones V Congreso Nacional del Laboratorio Clínico* 2011 (4) 190.

Martos, S. (2012) *Comunidades de práctica. Cómo compartir conocimiento y experiencias profesionales*. Barcelona: UOC.

Mattoo, K., Mahajan, P. and Gaba, N. (2014) Surrogate request for visual brand identification for a completely edentulous patient with dementia. *American Journal of Medical Case Reports* 2 (9), 194–197.

Morales, O. (2010) *Los géneros escritos en la odontologia hispanoamericana. Estructuración retórica y estratègies de atenuación en artículos de investigación, casos clínicos y artículos de revisión*. PhD Universitat Pompeu Fabra. See http://www.tdx.cat/bitstream/handle/10803/7577/tom.pdf?sequence=1 (accessed 11 January 2014).

Niero, N. (2008) *Il mix fraqualità e quantità nella ricerca sociale*. Verona: QuiEdit.

Pahta, P. (2006) 'This is very important': A corpus study of amplifiers in medical writing. In M. Gotti and F. Salager-Mayer (eds) *Advances in Medical Discourse Analysis: Oral and Written Contexts* (pp. 357–381). Bern: Peter Lang.

Parodi, G. (2010) *Academic and Professional Discourse Genres in Spanish*. Amsterdam/Philadelphia, PA: John Benjamins.

Paveau, M-A. (2006) *Les Prédiscours. Sens, mémoire, cognition*. Paris: Presses Sorbonne Nouvelle.

Piqué-Angordans, J. and Posteguillo, S. (2006) Peer positive and negative assessment in medical English medical genres. In M. Gotti and F. Salager-Mayer (eds) *Advances in Medical Discourse Analysis: Oral and Written Contexts* (pp. 382–405). Bern: Peter Lang.

Reyes, N., Verduzco S., Sosa R., Zamora I., Guevara C., Contreras A., Martínez R., Galicia, A. and Varguéz, V. (2009) Ablación de vía accesoria lateral izquierda por punción transeptal en un paciente con síndrome de Wolf-Parkinson White y con problema de acceso arterial femoral. Presentación de un caso. *Archivos de Cardiología de México* 79 (1), 91–109.

Rodríguez, N. (2008) *Manual de sociología de las profesiones*. Barcelona: Publicaciones de la Universitat de Barcelona.

Rodríguez-Merchán, E.C. (2005) La política editorial de los casos clínicos. *Revista Española de Cirugía Ortopédica y Traumatología* 49 (4), 241.

Sacks, O. (1985) *The Man Who Mistook His Wife for a Hat*. London: Picador.

Salvador, V. (2015) Un nuevo modelo de discurso biográfico: los casos clínicos literaturizados de Oliver Sacks. In E. Balaguer, M.J. Francés and V. Vidal (eds) *Aproximació al'altre: biografies, semblances i retrats* (pp. 9–16). Amsterdam/Philadelphia, PA: John Bemjamins.

Salvador, V. and Macián, C. (2009) Primera relación entre paciente y profesional de la salud. Rituales de interacción y estrategias discursivas en las primeras visitas al podólogo. *Estudos Linguisticos/LinguisticStudies* 3, 439–457.

Salvador, V., Macián, C. and Marín, M.J. (2013) La construcción de las profesiones sanitarias a través de las revistas especializadas. *Discurso & Sociedad* 7 (1), 73–96. See http://www.dissoc.org/ediciones/v07n01/DS7%281%29Salvador%20et%20al.pdf (accessed10 July 2014).

Scollon, R. (2008) *Analyzing Public Discourse: Discourse Analysis in the Making of Public Policy*. New York: Routledge.

Swales, J.M. (1990) *Genre Analysis: English in Academic and Research Settings*. Cambridge: Cambridge University Press.

Turk, U., Basol, G., Barutcuoglu, B., Sahin, F., Habif, S., Tarugi, P. and Bayindir, O. (2012) A 54-year-old diabetic man with low serum cholesterol. *Clinical Chemistry* 58 (5), 826–830.

Uribarri, I. (2004) La descripción científica y el caso clínico. *Oftalmológica Santa Lucia*, 3. http://www.hospitalsantalucia.com.ar/osl/osl11/descripcion_cientifica.htm (accessed 30 January 2015).

Weiss, G. and Wodak, R. (eds) (2003) *Critical Discourse Analysis: Theory and Interdisciplinarity*. Basingstoke: Palgrave MacMillan.

Wells, C.E., Moulin, C.J.A., Ethridge, P., Illman, N.A., Davies, E. and Zeman, A. (2014) Persistent psychogenic déjà vu: a case report. *Journal of Medical Case Reports* 8 (414), 1–4.

Wenger, E. (1998) *Communities of Practice: Learning, Meaning, and Identity*. Cambridge: Cambridge University Press.

Whiteside, S.P. and Abramowitz, J.S. (2006) Relapse following successful intensive treatment of pediatric obsessive-compulsive disorder. A case study. *Clinical Case Studies* 5 (6), 522–540.

4 Popular Science Articles vs Scientific Articles: A Tool for Medical Education

Begoña Bellés-Fortuño

During the 19th century, the need to make science more accessible to the public resulted in the emergence of a new type of written genre, the popular science article (PSA; Meadows, 1987). In this study, I will contrast the structure of scientific research articles (RAs) and PSAs as well as some linguistic features such as the use of discourse markers and evaluative language in both genres. Here, I analyse a corpus of four articles: two PSAs taken from one of the top ten websites on popular science called Science Daily and two scientific articles published in a prestigious medical journal, The Lancet. The topic in the articles is the same: arthritis. To be able to compare and contrast the articles more effectively, corpus analysis tools have been used to analyse the linguistic features mentioned above. This chapter aims at showing how PSAs can be used as pedagogical material for the teaching of medicine, as they are more easily understandable for students (Parkinson & Adendorff, 2004), thereby providing a more intuitive learning process. On the other hand, scientific articles are a source of medical knowledge and should be taken into consideration accordingly. However, medical students in their first years at university who have never been exposed to academic and scientific articles may find the reading and understanding of this academic type of written genre difficult and arduous.

Introduction

Academic writing is a means of communication of a scientific community that uses the same scientific discourse. As Widdowson (1979: 52) claims, scientific discourse 'is realized by a scientific text in different languages by the process of textualization'. Thus, academia has taken the research article (RA) as the genre to spread knowledge and reach different audiences. Hyland (2010: 117) defines the RA as 'the principal site of disciplinary knowledge-making', or in Montgomery's (1996) words 'the master narrative of our time'. Swales (1990: 93) adds to the definition of an RA that 'it is to appear or has appeared in a research journal or, less typically, in an edited book-length collection of papers'. Therefore, the scientific RA has clearly identified writing conventions and norms, being primarily addressed to experts within a concrete scientific community or to a professional audience.

During the 19th century, the need to make science more accessible to a non-specialist public in the field enabled the onset of a new type of written genre, the popular science article (PSA) (Meadows, 1987). This need has been increasingly growing with the emergence of new technologies, their immediacy and rapid spread of knowledge. Nowadays, most daily newspapers have specialised science sections that are largely read (Pellechia, 1997) and the number of science articles in the press, on paper or in online format is constantly increasing.

The PSA can be addressed to a less expert audience; it provides readable and constant information in an easily accessible way. Popularisation is targeted to a wide reading public, although dealing with specialised topics; it is not addressed to an expert group but to a socially experienced audience (Gotti, 2014). In Hyland's (2010: 118) words, popular science 'is produced for audiences without a professional need for information about science but who want to keep abreast of developments'.

Academics should be aware of the different scientific discourses and how these affect and modulate the relations between science and society. In the discourse of popularisation, scientists often include views that may not derive from scientific sources and therefore generate an interest in the relation between science and society (Whitley, 1985). In terms of socio-economic impact, science is probably the fastest 'growing enterprise in our society' (Weingart, 2002: 703). Authors such as Weingart (2002) talk about a new phenomenon of 'growth-driven specialisation of science' that expands to society and to a wide variety of fields of study. He continues with a very illustrative metaphorical image of scientific knowledge by saying: 'Knowledge, as it enters the public arena, is inevitably judged and valued by society' (Weingart, 2002: 704). The link between science and society in our century is thus undeniable. In Gotti's words, the popularisation of science is an attempt to come closer to society.

> Viewed from this new perspective, popularization often provides explanations in terms of the social meaning of the events in question, which is indicative of an increased social awareness of risks (…) Rather than 'explaining science', this new type of popularization sets out to explain the social meaning of such events, with the consequent creation of interdiscursive texts mixing informative and explanatory

discourse with other scientifically-unrelated matters of more general public concern. (Gotti, 2014: 27)

Some studies have argued that PSAs cannot primarily serve as models for scientific writing (Parkinson & Adendorff, 2004); however, in my view, they can make science more accessible to undergraduate students in tertiary education. I believe that PSAs could be used as pedagogical tools in the university classroom to facilitate students' understanding of content.

The university classroom situation in the field of health sciences in Europe has changed over the last 10 years to adapt to the demands of the European Commission and the creation of the European Higher Education Area (EHEA) in accordance with the London Communiqué (2007). The European Commission, in successive meetings and plans (Commission of the European Communities: Action Plan 2004–2006), has emphasised the concept of 'employability' and foreign language learning as important aspects of degrees; universities should offer degrees that facilitate, as one of the main outcomes, graduate and postgraduate students' access to the professional world. Thus, there is a need to prepare health sciences students as professionals in a globalised world, where not only the specific contents of the field but also the learning of second or foreign languages are paramount for the construction of a dynamic tertiary education. Multilingual education constitutes a common goal of the European Union, where the English language has reached an overwhelming dominance as a lingua franca.

If we look at English for academic purposes (EAP) settings or at English for specific purposes (ESP) courses at any European or American university, what we can find is a group of non-native students who are enrolled in health sciences degrees where most or part of the tuition is delivered in English. In these higher education contexts, PSAs might become an extremely useful and illuminating tool for university students who are neither familiar with the academic genres nor used to receiving a large part or all of their lectures in a second or foreign language, especially in their first years at university. Content lecturers can facilitate their native or non-native students' subject content learning and on the other hand, English language lecturers can make the English language more comprehensible to their EAP or ESP university students.

It is largely known that the reading and understanding of a medical RA can be arduous for a non-expertise audience such as students in tertiary education, in particular during their first years of study. Clearly, RAs have an easily identifiable and conventionalised structure which has largely been analysed and discussed: introduction, method, results and discussion (Hyon, 1996; Swales, 1990). PSAs, on the contrary, seem not to have such a fixed standardised structure and organisation of information. They tend to adapt to the communication media where they are published, popular magazine or journal, on paper or online. However, there seems to be an agreement on how to present and organise information within the same communication channel in PSAs, something similar to a macrostructure of the genre, as I will explain later in this chapter.

RAs use forms of high formal register of language, technical lexicon, nominalisation, passivisation and impersonal tone (Parkinson & Adendorff, 2004) because they are addressed to a skilled and expert audience with a high level of expertise on the topic. As a consequence, the RA writer tries to mitigate the impact of what is being told by using hedging. On the contrary, PSAs 'show solidarity with the reader through treating the scientist participants as personalities, by humour, and, if the projected readers are non-scientists, by distancing the reader and writer from scientists as a group' (Parkinson & Adendorff, 2004: 389). That is, PSAs tend to use more informal language in a more direct way, sometimes including conversational style, which makes them suitable as an introductory reading on a specific scientific topic. These traits make the PSA a potential pedagogical tool for the university classroom without disregarding the more standardised academic article.

In the sections that follow, I aim at showing how the less conventionalised structure and less formal use of language of PSAs make them suitable models for teaching undergraduate students in the field of health sciences, especially those in the first year of their degree, whether native or non-native English students.

The Study

The study aims at analysing evaluative language and other linguistic features such as discourse markers (DMs) in terms of frequency of use and concordance occurrences (collocates) in order to identify, measure and analyse the evaluations and interactions that occur between writer and reader in health sciences academic writing in two different genres, medical RAs and PSAs. In an attempt to facilitate content acquisition for students of medicine, whether native or non-native in English, I intend to show that the PSA can be a central pedagogical tool for lecturers in the health sciences field, a means for a more comprehensible transmission of knowledge and thoughts in the tertiary education classroom.

The study of evaluative language in scientific and academic texts is not new. Although largely studied, evaluative language has always aroused discrepancies regarding the nature of evaluative features in discourse. Already in 1997, Thetela (1997: 102) stated that there was 'a lack of consensus among researchers on which lexical items are evaluative'. Here, I do not aim at providing a categorisation of evaluative language items and features in academic scientific writing as other studies and authors have already done (Bellés-Fortuño & Querol-Julián, 2010; Hyland, 1998, 1999, 2000, 2001, 2005; Oakey, 2005; Stotesbury, 2003; Webber, 2004; among others). The main objective is to detect recurrent evaluative language patterns in RAs and PSAs in order to observe similarities or differences between these two genres and to understand the way these evaluative language items behave and make the texts comprehensible to the audience.

Evaluation is a means of interaction between writer and reader. In this study, evaluative language in academic discourse is understood as 'the expression of the speaker or writer's attitude or stance towards, viewpoint on, or feelings about entities or propositions that he or she is talking about' (Thompson & Hunston, 2000: 5). In this line, this study aims at detecting and analysing explicit evaluation forms of attitudinal language disregarding forms of implicit evaluation; the latter is assumed to be the most commonly used evaluation in academic texts (Hunston, 1993, 1994). By analysing the use of evaluative language in two different academic genres (RAs and PSAs), the particular interpersonal negotiations established between writers and readers in scientific literacy can be observed.

As for DMs, they have largely proven their effectiveness for the comprehension of connected discourse (Bellés-Fortuño, 2008; Chaudron & Richards, 1986; Cook, 1975; Kinstch & Yarbrough, 1982; Murphy & Candlin, 1979). Most researchers agree on the underlying concept of DMs, although these have taken different names: cue phrases (Knott & Dale, 1994), discourse connectives (Redeker, 1990), pragmatic markers (Fraser, 1988, 1999; Schiffrin, 1987), among other terms.

Here, I take the view of researchers such as Schiffrin (1987) and Fraser (1999, 2004), who approach DMs from a grammatical-pragmatic perspective, both agreeing on DMs as having a core meaning. Fraser (2004) distinguishes among syntactic, semantic and pragmatic properties of DMs, differentiating categories within these three properties. Following his approach, DMs, in this chapter, are defined as:

> A class of lexical expressions drawn primarily from the syntactic classes of conjunctions, adverbs and prepositional phrases. With certain exceptions, they signal a relationship between the interpretation of the segment they introduce, S2, and the prior segment, S1. (Fraser, 1999: 937)

Following Fraser's (2004) classification of DMs according to syntactic categories such as coordinate conjunctions, subordinate conjunctions, adverbials, prepositional phrases and prepositions, I will try to identify frequent uses of DMs in the corpus. This classification, although useful for a first identification, may fail in categorising some cases of markers; therefore, a second, more complex classification of DMs, also proposed by Fraser (2004) and based on semantic relationships, where categories such as contrastive, elaborative, implicative or temporal markers are included, will be taken into consideration for the analysis of the corpus.

A combination of these two classifications proposed by Fraser (2004) seems logical for the analysis of the corpus under study, while the syntactic categories will help to identify the most distinctive markers, the marginal classification based on semantic categories will also allow me to explain some other pragmatic examples of DMs that may appear in the corpus, especially in Corpus B including examples of PSAs, a less conventionalised and standardised genre.

The analysis that follows presents a contrastive genre analysis of two academic written genres (RAs and PSAs) in the field of health sciences. I aim at identifying, observing and analysing differences and/or similarities in the use of some evaluative language items and DMs according to recurrent use as well as some marginal uses of collocational patterns in both types of text. The study departs from the following questions: (a) Do cohesive devices such as DMs differ in type and frequency between RAs and PSAs? and (b) Is language use more evaluative in one of these two genres? If so, how can this affect the way that readers process information?

By looking into these features, I intend to present PSAs as a more understandable and comprehensible type of text or genre (both terms interchangeable here) for university students in the field of health sciences. PSAs could therefore be used as classroom materials in the English for health sciences classroom, motivating students and enhancing a more successful acquisition of content and language.

Method

The corpus

To carry out the analysis, I have compiled a corpus of four articles in total; the first two articles, which will be referred to as Corpus A, are two scientific RAs published in a prestigious medical journal, *The Lancet*; Corpus B comprises two PSAs taken from one of the top ten websites on popular science named *Science Daily*. The topic of the articles included in the corpus is the same for the four of them: arthritis; this makes it possible to compare how the message is transmitted from writer to reader in both genres. The data sample analysed permits the realisation of a small corpus study.

The whole corpus (Corpus A plus Corpus B), although not too large in number of articles, has proven to be a valid sample for the analysis of the different uses of DMs and some evaluative language tokens as explained in the previous section. Tables 4.1 and 4.2 provide more detailed information about the four articles (ARs) included in the corpus, their titles and the total number of words. RAs, as well as being a more conventionalised genre, are longer texts. Neither of the *Science Daily* PSAs exceed 1500 words.

There is a longer tradition of studying and analysing RAs, in which a fixed macrostructure has been identified; this macrostructure appears to occur irrespective of the field they belong to. When examining Corpus B, one can also discern a regular macrostructure in the PSAs corpus from *Science*

Table 4.1 Description of the four articles (ARs) included in the total corpus and the total number of words

Code	*Source*	*Title*	*No. words*
AR1	*The Lancet*	Rheumatoid arthritis	6,444
AR2	*The Lancet*	Efficacy and safety of leflunomide compared with placebo and sulphasalazine in active rheumatoid arthritis	6,353
AR3	*Science Daily*	Drivers of rheumatoid arthritis identified	1,121
AR4	*Science Daily*	Hip replacement an excellent option for young juvenile arthritis patients	1,420
Total			15,338

Daily, a structure that seems to resemble that of RAs, but it is simpler and more visual. This fact is not surprising, since *Science Daily* publishes online and fits to the conventions of the web genres, where visual material is a key factor for attracting the reader.

Science Daily is advertised as a source for the latest research news that presents featured research. The word *research* is recurrent throughout the site in order to differentiate it from tabloids or other types of web press. *Science Daily* web articles include a main title, date of publication, source and a summary that resembles *The Lancet* abstract but is shorter in length (see Appendices 1 and 2 for samples of Corpus A and Corpus B); both genres share the same initial information and structure. It is worth mentioning one special feature that those articles in Corpus B share. At the end of these articles, the *Science Daily* site offers different formats for the citation of the respective articles in a highly standardised scientific way. The three main citation styles for research are hyperlinked: Modern Language Association (MLA), American Psychological Association (APA) and Chicago styles are available just by clicking on them (see Figure 4.1).

Having presented the main features and utility of the two corpora under study, in the following section, I will describe the method of analysis used in order to observe some differences and/or similarities between RAs and PSAs in the use and treatment of evaluative tokens and some linguistics features. The analysis will try to support the initial hypothesis that health

Table 4.2 Total number of words per corpus (Corpus A and Corpus B)

	Total no. Words
Corpus A (RAs)	12,797w
Corpus B (PSAs)	2,541w

Cite this page:

- MLA
- APA
- Chicago

Hospital for Special Surgery. "Hip replacement an excellent option for young juvenile arthritis patients." Science Daily. ScienceDaily, 17 November 2014. <www.sciencedaily.com/releases/2014/11/141117093332.htm>.

Figure 4.1 Example of hyperlinked citation styles in AR4 (Corpus B). The citation shown corresponds to MLA style

sciences PSAs could be a more appropriate type of text for undergraduate students and should be included as part of class material for the teaching of medical concepts in English native or non-native learning settings and, more specifically, to university students in their first years of medicine studies.

The analysis

For the analysis of the corpus, the online Lextutor v.8 (Cobb, 2002; Heatley *et al.*, 2002) search tool was used. Lextutor is a powerful online search tool to analyse the use of specific words in English texts. Among other procedures, it allows the user to copy and paste shorter texts to be analysed, as well as to upload the user's own corpus, provided that it does not exceed 4MB. The latter option was chosen for the current analysis. Lextutor v.8 is able to extract basic frequency lists and select recurrent words (word extractor) (see Table 4.3). It is also a very powerful online concordancer that allows users to identify collocational patterns in their own corpora and establish patterns of use.

For the analysis, I firstly conducted a search in both corpora (Corpus A and Corpus B) in order to get frequency lists of words. The lists obtained served to detect the use of DMs in both corpora. A closer look at the frequency list gave us an approximation of the type and number of uses of DMs in both corpora (Corpus A and Corpus B) following Fraser's (1999, 2004) study on DMs.

The same procedure was used for the analysis of evaluative tokens. The frequency lists obtained served as a guidance to extract those most recurrent evaluative tokens in Corpus A and Corpus B, by taking into consideration explicit forms of evaluation in attitudinal language (Thompson & Hunston, 2000). As usual in corpus linguistic analyses, the data extracted automatically are of great help for the study; nevertheless, individual cases were hand-edited and examined in a much more detailed way.

For both searches (DMs and evaluative tokens), the previous studies already mentioned in this chapter (Fraser, 1999, 2004; Hunston, 1993;

Table 4.3 Partial sample of the frequency list of AR3 extracted from Lextutor v.8

Rank	*Freq*	*Coverage individ/cumulative*		*Word*
1.	30	5.06%	5.06%	THE
2.	21	3.54%	8.60%	TO
3.	19	3.20%	11.80%	AND
4.	18	3.04%	14.84%	IN
5.	14	2.36%	17.20%	OF
6.	11	1.85%	19.05%	RA
7.	10	1.69%	20.74%	CELLS
8.	10	1.69%	22.43%	PEOPLE
9.	10	1.69%	24.12%	THAT
10.	9	1.52%	25.64%	A

Schiffrin, 1987; Thompson & Hunston, 2000) were extremely useful, particularly due to their attempts to elaborate open classifications and categories of these linguistic features.

An exhaustive analysis of the two corpora was firstly conducted with the help of Lextutor; the preliminary results were then checked and proofread within the context of the original texts. The initial data obtained were later used for a deeper qualitative analysis within the generic corpus context, combining both empirical and hermeneutic approaches.

Results

The findings are presented in order, beginning with the results obtained after analysing DMs, followed by evaluative tokens. Though not one of the main objectives of this study, some observations regarding evident patterns of collocation will also be made; only significant instances will be mentioned.

DMs results

The most frequently used DMs in Corpus A (RAs) are, in order of frequency: *however, although, furthermore, then, because of, therefore, despite, thus, in addition* and *by contrast*. *However, although,* and *furthermore* are the three most recurrent ones with 19, 12 and 10 instances, respectively. *Therefore, despite* and *thus* share the same number of instances (4) as well as *in addition* and *by contrast* with three instances each (see Table 4.4 and the following examples).

Table 4.4 Most frequently used DMs in Corpus A

Position	*DMs*	*No. occurrences*	*‰*
1	*however*	19	1.4
2	*although*	12	0.9
3	*furthermore*	10	0.8
4	*then*	9	0.7
5	*because of*	5	0.4
6	*therefore*	4	0.3
7	*despite*	4	0.3
8	*thus*	4	0.3
9	*in addition*	3	0.3
10	*by contrast*	3	0.3

(1) A recent investigation found consistent use of DMARDs in patients with moderate or long-standing rheumatoid arthritis. **However**, only a few DMARDs have been unequivocally shown to retard radiographically assessed disease progression; sulphasalazine is one of these DMARDs. (AR2/Corpus A)

(2) Leflunomide is an orally available inhibitor of dihydro-orotate dehydrogenase–an enzyme required for de-novo pyrimidine synthesis. **Although** its specific mechanism of action in rheumatoid arthritis is not known, leflunomide affects lymphocyte function in vivo and in vitro. (AR1/Corpus A)

(3) The corresponding rates for a 50% improvement in ACR score were 34% and 33% at 24 and 52 weeks for leflunomide, and 8% and 14% for placebo. **Furthermore**, other studies showed that leflunomide slowed the progression of joint destruction and improved functional status and quality of life. (AR1/Corpus A)

As seen in Examples 1, 2 and 3, Corpus A tends to use DMs that fall into the categories of Contrastive (*however, although*) and Elaborative (*furthermore*) rather than Implicative (*because of, therefore*) or Temporal (*then*), that are also used but less frequently.

In Corpus B, the most recurrent DMs are, in order of frequency: *but, although, in addition, as a result, for the first time, the next step* and *in the long term* among others, *but* and *although* being the most recurrent ones with five and four instances, respectively. The rest of the DMs used only occur once each in the entire Corpus B. In this case, the most recurrent DMs in Corpus B fall into the Contrastive category; there are also examples of the other categories such as Implicative (*as a result*), Temporal (*for the first*

Table 4.5 Most frequently used DMs in Corpus B

Position	*DMs*	*No. occurrences*	*‰*
1	*but*	5	1.9
2	*although*	4	1.5
3	*in addition*	1	0.4
4	*as a result*	1	0.4
5	*for the first time of*	1	0.4
6	*the next step*	1	0.4
7	*in the long term*	1	0.4

time, the next step) and Elaborative (*in addition*) but with a lower number of instances (see Table 4.5 and the following examples).

(4) 'The surgery in this patient population, **although** performed by only a small number of specialized orthopaedic surgeons nationwide, is life-changing for JIA patients' said Mark P. Figgie M.D., senior author of the study and chief of the Surgical Arthritis Service at HSS. (AR4/Corpus B)

(5) If people are appropriately diagnosed and treated, they can work full time and be healthy, active adults. **But** they can still suffer and need medications that have risks and side effects. (AR3/Corpus B)

(6) Rheumatoid arthritis is thought to be a T cell mediated disease and is caused when the body's immune system mistakenly begins to attack its own tissues, primarily the synovium, the membrane that lines the joints. **As a result** of this autoimmune response, fluid builds up in the joins, causing joint pain and systematic inflammation. (AR3/Corpus B)

It is worth mentioning that in Corpus B there seems to be a higher use of DMs when a quotation occurs, the majority of the DMs used occur embedded in first-person quotes as seen in Example 4. The use of first-person quotes is a defining characteristic of PSAs.

Evaluative tokens results

Evaluative tokens as forms of attitudinal language used to convey writer and reader's interpersonal communication are highly frequent in the corpus under study. The evaluative features identified in the corpus have proven to have a relevance-signalling function linking the text and the audience, and among these features adjectives of relevance are particularly noteworthy. The top ten most recurrent evaluative items in Corpus A (RAs) are primarily adjectives and adverbs, as can be seen in Table 4.6.

Table 4.6 Most frequently used evaluative tokens in Corpus A

Position	*Evaluative token*	*No. occurrences*	*‰*
1	*high* (21) – *higher* (7)	28	2.2
2	*more+adj.*	16	1.2
3	*significant* (8) – *significantly* (7)	15	1.1
4	*rapid* (11) – *rapidly* (4)	15	1.1
5	*substantial*	13	1.0
6	*poor* (8) – *poorly* (2)	10	0.7
7	*progressive*	8	0.6
8	*serious*	7	0.5
9	*severe*	5	0.4
10	*aggressive*	3	0.2

The most frequently used evaluative items in Corpus A are the adjective *high*, also used in the comparative form (*higher*), followed by the combination of the comparative adverb *more+adjective* (*+than*) and the adjective *significant* and also its adverbial form *significantly*, sharing a number of instances with the adjective *rapid* and its adverbial form *rapidly* (see Examples 7, 8 and 9). There are other adjectives that usually appear in their positive form, for example, *substantial* and *progressive* with a relatively high number of instances (see Examples 10 and 11).

(7) There were two cases of reversible agranulocytosis in the sulphasalazine group. Interpretation Leflunomide was **more effective** than placebo in treatment of rheumatoid arthritis and showed similar efficacy to sulphasalazine. (Corpus A/AR2)

(8) These findings are the consequences of progressive disease, and have provided the impetus for development of **more effective** therapies to prevent joint destruction and maintain functional status. (Corpus A/AR1)

(9) Metalloproteinases are produced at **high** levels by type B synoviocytes in rheumatoid arthritis. Metalloproteinases are a family of enzymes required for remodelling and destruction of extracellular matrix. (Corpus A/AR1)

(10) We emphasise that these results should be interpreted with caution, since radiographs were missing for **substantial** numbers of patients, and the frequencies of American College of Rheumatology response rates were higher among patients with available radiographs than among those with missing radiographs in all three treatment groups. (Corpus A/AR2)

(11) The predominant symptoms are pain, stiffness, and swelling of peripheral joints (panel 1). The clinical course of the disorder is extremely variable, ranging from mild, self-limiting arthritis to rapidly **progressive** multisystem inflammation with profound morbidity and mortality (panel 2). Analyses of the clinical course and of laboratory and radiological abnormalities have defined negative prognostic factors for **progressive** joint destruction (panel 3). (Corpus A/AR1)

A closer look was taken at these evaluative items using the text-based Lextutor concordance tool in an attempt to identify any collocational pattern occurrences among the previously identified evaluative tokens. The search revealed that most occurrences of the grammatical pattern *more+adjective* (*+than*) were the combination of the adverb *more* plus the adjective *effective*, which semantically conveys a positive message for the reader, as can be seen in Examples 7 and 8.

Another pattern identified as a collocational pattern is the use of the adjective *significant* and its adverbial variation *significantly*, co-occurring usually with verbs or adjectives that implicitly express numerical or statistical data, introducing accurate figures, as shown in Examples 12 and 13.

(12) Hence, the limitation of the acute- phase response is an integral component of activity criteria in rheumatoidarthritis and response criteria for efficacy of DMARDs Leflunomide treatment was associated with **significant** decreases in CRP and ESR. However, the fall in ESR was **much less** pronounced than that in CRP. (Corpus A/AR2)

(13) Leflunomide and sulphasalazine were **significantly** superior to placebo ($p=0.0001$ for joint counts; $p<0.001$ for assessments). Radiographic disease progression was **significantly** slower with leflunomide and sulphasalazine than with placebo ($p<0.01$). (Corpus A/AR2)

As for Corpus B (PSAs), the evaluative tokens observed highlighted some recurrent evaluative adjectives and adverbs. The three most frequently used evaluative items are the adjectives *excellent*, followed by *severe* (or its adverbial form *severely*) and *unique*.

More adverbs have been used, such as *nearly* or *permanently*, along with others that have not been included in Table 4.7 because they do not have a high number of instances.

The adjective *excellent* ranks first in the list with a total number of five instances. A closer look at the contextual elements that co-occur with

Table 4.7 Most frequently used evaluative tokens in Corpus B

Position	*Evaluative token*	*No. occurrences*	*‰*
1	*excellent*	5	1.9
2	*severe* (2) – *severely* (1)	3	1.2
3	*unique*	2	0.8
4	*nearly*	2	0.8
5	*permanently*	1	0.4

the adjective *excellent* reveals a repetitive collocational pattern with the combination of *excellent* plus the noun *option* or the nouns *treatment option* (see Examples 14 and 15). This adverb is in fact included in the title of one of the ARs and is generally repeated throughout the text.

(14) Total hip replacement is an **excellent** option for patients under age 35 when conservative treatments fail to provide pain relief, researchers have found. The implant lasted at least 10 years in 85 percent of patients. (Corpus B/AR4)

(15) 'We concluded that overall, hip replacement is an **excellent** treatment option for young JIA patients with reasonable long-term implant survival and favorable patient-reported outcomes after surgery,' Dr. Swarup said. Although a good treatment, Dr. Figgie noted that the longevity of the implants needs to be improved, especially since the patients are so young. (Corpus B/AR4)

The second most frequent evaluative token in Corpus B is the adjective *severe* and the corresponding adverb *severely*, forms that, when contextualised, generally convey a negative meaning (*severely damaged*, *severe disease*, *severe joint deformities*). The use of comparative forms of the adjective in Corpus B is less frequent than in Corpus A; the scarce instances of comparatives found in Corpus B usually co-occur with other comparative or intensified forms to strengthen the meaning of the adjective that they accompany, as shown in Example 16, where the comparative *adverb* more semantically reinforces the adverse meaning of the adjective *severe*. There are other adverbs that semantically reinforce the meaning of the noun or adjective they accompany (see underlined instances in Examples 16 and 18).

(16) 'We were not surprised that the patients who received custom implants had lower scores since the very fact that they needed a custom implant meant they had more **severe** joint deformities and more **severe** disease,' Dr. Figgie explained. (AR4/Corpus B)

Although an adjective ranks highest in the list of the most frequently used evaluative tokens in Corpus B, a more general view of the evaluative items shows that adverbs are also of relevance in Corpus B, especially when compared to Corpus A, which contains a higher number of evaluative adjectives. Thus, other adverbs such as *nearly, permanently, mistakenly, especially, recently* and *primarily* are largely used throughout Corpus B, clarifying or adding precise meaning to the verbs they accompany.

(17) An estimated 1.3 million people in the United States have RA – almost 1 percent of the nation's adult population. There are **nearly** three times as many women as men with the disease. In women, RA most commonly begins between the ages of 30 and 60. (AR3/Corpus B)

(18) The drugs can be costly and sometimes they don't work or eventually stop working. If untreated, the disease will **permanently** destroy joints and cause pain. (AR3/Corpus B)

(19) Rheumatoid arthritis is thought to be a T cell mediated disease and is caused when the body's immune system **mistakenly** begins to attack its own tissues, **primarily** the synovium, the membrane that lines the joints. (AR3/Corpus B)

After having observed and analysed instances of DMs and evaluative language tokens in a very detailed way, comparing both subcorpora (Corpus A and Corpus B), in the next section a general comparative overview of the features analysed and the results obtained are presented.

Results overview

As a general overview of the whole corpus and in an attempt to compare Corpus A (RAs) and Corpus B (PSAs) concerning the use and frequency of DMs and evaluative tokens, the results have shown that PSAs (Corpus B) tend to use slightly more DMs than RAs. Although not a significant difference, the result in Corpus B is slightly higher. It has also been observed that Corpus A and Corpus B share some DMs used, especially those within the Contrastive category such as *although*. However, there seems to be a distinguishing trait regarding the form of DMs; the DMs used in Corpus B are not isolated forms of language such as *however, although* or *furthermore*, which are definitely quite common in Corpus A, but longer phrases and expressions that sometimes introduce direct speech quotes. Ultimately, Contrastive and Elaborative markers seem to be extensively used in both RAs and PSAs to express meaning and transmit information to the reader. These two categories stand out, followed by other categories such as Implicative, Elaborative or Temporal with less frequency of use.

Table 4.8 Overview results of Corpus A and Corpus B: DMs and evaluative tokens

	DMs	*Total (‰)*	*Evaluative tokens*	*Total (‰)*
Corpus A (RAs)	64	5.0	109	8.5
Corpus B (PSAs)	13	5.5	35	13.8

Regarding the use of explicit evaluative tokens, PSAs (Corpus B) have proven to use more evaluative language than Corpus A (RAs), despite being shorter, less extensive and grammatically simpler texts. The total average use of explicit evaluative items in Corpus B is 13.8% compared to a lower 8.5% in Corpus A (see Table 4.8), which reveals the emphasis on interpersonal communication in the text. The forms of explicit evaluative language found seem to differ slightly between Corpus A and Corpus B. Whereas Corpus A usually uses comparative forms of the adjective to convey evaluation, Corpus B combines the use of adjectives and adverbs, the latter being extensively used throughout the corpus, while comparative and superlative forms of adjectives are scarce.

Conclusions

Conclusions to this study can be drawn in two different dimensions. On the one hand, the exploration of some concrete linguistics features along with the text and context relations as they occur in two different academic genres (RAs and PSAs) and the interpersonal relations between writer and reader have been observed. On the other hand, a study like the one presented here allows us to draw some conclusions as to the practical purpose and the function of the genres under study, their practices and value in different settings and discourse communities. Small corpora studies such as the one carried out here allow a more qualitative interpretation of data and a deeper analysis of the genre texts as opposed to other large corpora studies whose findings are often exclusively based on a large amount of data.

Formal remarks

This study departed from the following research questions: (a) Do cohesive devices such as DMs differ in type and frequency between RAs and PSAs? and (b) Is language use more evaluative in one of these two genres? If so, how can this affect the way that readers process information? The conclusions drawn from the analysis show that DMs in PSAs are slightly higher in frequency than in RAs, which implies a higher degree of text organisation and therefore a clearer guidance for the reader, which ultimately generates a deeper comprehension of the text. The types of DMs used in PSAs are not exclusively fixed isolated forms of connectors, as is the case in RA texts, but rather prepositional phrases or noun phrases, more typical forms of spoken academic discourse, which involves a lower degree of language formality and a less formal register. Both genres (RAs and PSAs) produce a coherent discourse thanks to the use of DMs and both convey meaning mainly by comparing and contrasting ideas, as the findings have shown.

In popular science texts, human participants play an important role and, as a consequence, the use of direct speech quotations is common. In the voices of human participants, the use of DMs resembles spontaneous spoken discourse. These expressions of personal attitudes affect the use of evaluative items. The study has shown that evaluative language is more relevant in PSAs. This is the result of a particular focus on the people engaged in the research rather than on the analysis and the processes involved. As a result, PSAs are less impersonal and have a higher degree of subjectivity, focusing on human participants, their thoughts and beliefs, thereby creating bond between writer and reader's interpersonal communication. The interpersonal relations created between writer and reader are the result of evaluative language use. In the corpus under study, PSAs have proven to use a higher number of evaluative tokens than Corpus A (RAs) by using adjectives and especially adverbs to position the reader in the texts and direct him/her towards the ideas shown. In both corpora, writers have been very careful about lexical accuracy; adjectives and adverbs are sharp and strict, and there is no room for misunderstandings or different gradations. Adjectives are 'straight to the point' and that is the way readers interpret them (see Examples 7, 10, 11, 14 and 16). The writer's task is more complex than simply choosing which adjective or adverb is contextually accurate or conveys a meaning established for a specific group of users or discourse community (the scientific community in this case); writers aim at *lexical acuity*, a concept I use here to refer to the writer's precise evaluation of what is being said and his/her ability to create interpersonal relations with the reader through explanation and expository clarity.

Having seen this, one may think that PSAs are very distant from academic research writing. This idea is far from reality: popularisation is just another type of written academic genre, and it shares some traits with RA writing such as the use of specific and technical vocabulary, similar structure of the text and the fact that both genres are always related to a scientific topic. *Science Daily*, one of the most well-known and read popular science websites presents itself as 'Your source for the latest research news' and displays what it calls 'Featured research', emphasising that what the reader can find there is scientific research. As already mentioned in this chapter, the *Science Daily* website includes a hyperlinked section to help the reader in case he/she needs to reference the article. The reader is provided, just by a quick click of the mouse, with the article referenced in the three most standardised scientific ways of citing: APA, MLA and Chicago citation styles. This fact contradicts some previous studies which claimed that PSAs cite references in a popular rather than an academic style (Parkinson & Adendorff, 2004).

The truth is that health sciences research is very dynamic and constantly evolving (Gil-Salom, 2001) in such a rapid way, and with such a massive amount of information for the scientific community, that it can be hard for a researcher to keep constantly updated with the latest advances in medicine. In this respect, popular articles give the scientific community a chance to easily grasp the latest advances and research in medicine in a simpler and more accessible way. The question, therefore, is: why not use PSAs as pedagogical tools for undergraduate students? As discussed in this chapter, on the whole, PSAs have here proven to be a less standardised and more persuasive genre, with less-established norms but are well-organised and easier to comprehend.

Pedagogical reflections

PSAs in the health sciences field have proven to be simpler and shorter texts compared to medical RAs. These factors make them less difficult to read and easier to understand, that is why they are quite a suitable first reading and introduction to a medical topic for university students, especially in their first years, who are not yet familiar or acquainted with the conventions of scientific academic writing. An easier and clearer understanding and comprehension of PSAs in the classroom avoids rejection of the use of a foreign language in the educational setting for non-native students who have to study and use English as a vehicular language in the tertiary classroom in the medical field.

Non-native health sciences university students find themselves helpless when having to read and discuss, in class, a scientific RA published in a prestigious journal. Most lecturers believe that exposing students to original RAs in the English language is a good learning practice. However, during my years of experience as a lecturer of English for health sciences, I have observed that novel university students (especially those in their first and second years at university) find the reading and comprehension of academic RAs dull, confusing and hard to understand. The fact is that they have not been exposed to this kind of academic literacy in secondary schools, not even to academic texts in their mother tongues. Accordingly, they are not familiar with the conventions of the genre in the native languages and they can very hardly be familiar with this type of text in a foreign language like English. Most Spanish university lecturers tend to forget that the level of a foreign language such as English among health sciences tertiary students when entering university is far from homogeneous; very few students reach or are above the intermediate B2 level according to the Common European Framework for Language Reference (CEFR). This situation is typical of universities within the European Union that have made the language requirements of the European Commission mandatory and are now offering most of their degrees or part of the tuition of their degrees in English as the vehicular language. Obviously, the situation is not the same in every single country in the EU and depends on the level of exposure to the English language at early stages. However, this situation can also be extended to English-speaking countries and universities whose students have not been exposed to and taught the conventions of academic literacy before entering university in any field of knowledge and the medical field in the case under study.

As a consequence, introducing English health sciences PSAs in the university classroom and syllabus may not only enhance successful learning of contents, but it will also improve the learning of English as a second or foreign language in higher education, avoiding rejection and increasing motivation. The introduction and presentation in the classroom setting of lists of frequently used evaluative tokens and DMs, such as the ones identified in this study, and the creation of activities based on them, such as, for instance, the identification of language patterns in PSAs and the comparison with RAs, could be an example of a pedagogical proposal for the university classroom.

Thus, the findings derived from the current study can be very useful to develop pedagogical tools for the teaching of university students enrolled in health sciences degrees to write academic scientific texts. By means of comparing PSAs and RAs, students can learn about the differences between academic genres and improve their writing skills as future researchers and scientists in a particular scientific community. Native and non-native undergraduate students in the medical field as well as lecturers, also native or non-native, who have to deliver their lessons on medicine in English, can benefit from the results of this study, thus providing a further contribution to the broad and extensively studied field of EAP and the closely related field of ESP.

The present study has aimed at analysing in a broad sense the relations established in scientific writing, which have been observed and examined according to the following three main dimensions or scopes: (a) the relations in scientific writing between science and society; (b) the interpersonal relations established in academic written texts between writer and reader; and (c) the relations of the two genres (RAs and PSAs) regarding text and context. These relations are centred on the purpose of the genres analysed and the discourse communities involved and addressed. At a lower and closer level of analysis, the study has provided insights into the recurrent language patterns used in both written genres (RAs and PSAs).

References

Bellés-Fortuño, B. (2008) *A Spoken Academic Discourse Contrastive Study: Discourse Markers in North-American and Spanish Lectures*. Monográfico. Logroño: Revista de la Asociación Española de Lingüística Aplicada.

Bellés-Fortuño, B. and Querol Julián, M. (2010) Evaluation in research article abstracts: A cross-cultural study between Spanish and English medical discourse. In R. Lorés-Sanz, P. Mur-Dueñas and E. Lafuente-Millán (eds) *Constructing Interpersonality. Multiple Perspectives on Written Academic Genres* (pp. 83–98). Newcastle upon Tyne: Cambridge Scholars Publishing.

Chaudron, C. and Richards, J.C. (1986) The effect of discourse markers on the comprehension of lectures. *Applied Linguistics* 7, 113–127.

Cobb, T. (2002) *Web Vocabprofile*. See http://www.lextutor.ca/vp/ (accessed 21 January 2015); an adaptation of Heatley *et al.*'s (2002) range.

Commission of the European Communities: Action Plan 2004–2006. Communication from the Commission to the Council, the European Parliament, the Economic and Social Committee and the Committee of the Regions Promoting language learning and linguistic diversity. See http://europa.eu/legislation_summaries/education_training_youth/lifelong_learning/c11068_en.htm (accessed 21 January 2015).

Cook, J.R.S. (1975) A communicative approach to the analysis of extended monologue and its relevance to the development of teaching material for ESP. Unpublished PhD thesis, University of Edinburgh.

Fraser, B. (1988) Types of English discourse markers. *Acta Linguistica Hungarica* 38 (1–4), 19–33.

Fraser, B. (1999) What are discourse markers? *Journal of Pragmatics* 31, 931–952.

Fraser, B. (2004) An account of discourse markers. In P. Garcés, R. Gómez, L. Fernández and M. Padilla (eds) *Current Trends in Intercultural, Cognitive and Social Pragmatics* (pp. 13–34). Sevilla: Publicaciones de la Universidad de Sevilla.

Gil-Salom, L. (2001) El discurso de la ciencia y la tecnología: El artículo científico de investigación versus el artículo de divulgación científica. *Revista Española de Lingüística Aplicada* 14, 429–449.

Gotti, M. (2014) Reformulation and recontextualization in popularization discourse. *IBÉRICA* 27, 15–34.

Heatley, A., Nation, I.S.P. and Coxhead, A. (2002) RANGE and FREQUENCY programs. See http://www.victoria.ac.nz/lals/staff/paul-nation.aspx (accessed 21 January 2015).

Hunston, S. (1993) Evaluation and ideology in scientific writing. In M. Ghadessy (ed.) *Register Analysis: Theory and Practice* (pp. 57–73). London: Pinter.

Hunston, S. (1994) Evaluation and organization in a sample of written academic discourse. In M. Coulthard (ed.) *Advances in Written Text Analysis* (pp. 191–218). London: Routledge.

Hyland, K. (1998) Persuasion and context: The pragmatics of academic discourse. *Journal of Pragmatics* 30, 437–455.

Hyland, K. (1999) Disciplinary discourses: Writer stance in research articles. In C. Candlin and K. Hyland (eds) *Writing: Texts, Processes and Practices* (pp. 99–121). London: Longman.

Hyland, K. (2000) *Disciplinary Discourses: Social Interactions in Academic Writing*. London: Longman.

Hyland, K. (2001) Bringing the reader: Addressee features in academic articles. *Writing Communication* 18 (4), 549–574.

Hyland, K. (2005) Engagements and disciplinarity: The other side of evaluation. In G. Del Lungo Camiciotty and E. Tognini Bonelli (eds) *Academic Discourse: New Insights into Evaluation* (pp. 13–30). Bern: Peter Lang.

Hyland, K. (2010) Constructing proximity: Relating to readers in popular and professional science. *Journal of English for Academic Purposes* 9, 116–127.
Hyon, S (1996) Genre in the three traditions: Implications for ESL. *TESOL Quarterly* 30 (4), 693–722.
Kinstch, W. and Yarbrough, J.C. (1982) Role of rhetorical structure in text comprehension. *Journal of Educational Psychology* 74 (6), 828–834.
Knott, A. and Dale, R. (1994) Using linguistic phenomena to motivate a set of coherence relations. *Discourse Processes* 18 (1), 35–62.
London Communiqué (2007) Towards the European Higher Education Area: Responding to challenges in a globalized world. See https://www.eqar.eu/fileadmin/documents/bologna/London-Communique-18May2007.pdf (accessed 21 January 2015).
Meadows, J. (1987) The growth of science popularization: A historical sketch. *IMPACT of Science on Society* 144, 341–346.
Montgomery, S. (1996) *The Scientific Voice*. New York: The Guilford Press.
Murphy, D.F. and Candlin, C.N. (1979) Engineering lecture discourse and listening comprehension. *Practical Papers in English Language Education 2* (pp. 1–79). Lancaster: University of Lancaster.
Oakey, D. (2005) Academic vocabulary in academic discourse. The phraseological behaviour of EVALUATION in economics research articles. In E. Tognini Bonilli and G. Del Lungo Camiciotti (eds) *Strategies in Academic Discourse* (pp. 169–183). Amsterdam/Philadelphia, PA: John Benjamins.
Parkinson, J. and Adendorff, R. (2004) The use of popular science articles in teaching scientific literacy. *English for Specific Purposes* 23, 379–396.
Pellechia, M. (1997) Trends in science coverage: A content analysis of three US newspapers. *Public Understanding of Science* 6, 49–68.
Redeker, G. (1990) Ideational and pragmative markers of discourse structure. *Journal of Pragmatics* 14 (3), 367–381.
Schiffrin, D. (1987) *Discourse Markers*. Cambridge: Cambridge University Press.
Stotesbury, H. (2003) Evaluation in research article abstracts in the narrative and hard sciences. *Journal of English for Academic Purposes* 2, 327–341.
Swales, J.M. (1990) *Genre Analysis*. Cambridge: Cambridge University Press.
Thetela, P. (1997) Evaluated entities and parameters of value in academic research articles. *English for Specific Purposes* 16 (2), 101–118.
Thompson, G. and Hunston, S. (2000) Evaluation: An introduction. In S. Hunston and G. Thompson (eds) *Evaluation in Text: Authorial Stance and the Construction of Discourse* (pp. 1–27). Oxford: Oxford University Press.
Webber, P. (2004) Negotiation in linguistic papers. In G. Del Lungo Camiciotti and E. Tognini Bonilli (eds) *Academic Discourse: New Insights into Evaluation* (pp. 181–202). Bern: Peter Lang.
Weingart, P. (2002) The moment of truth for science: The consequences of the 'knowledge society' for society and science. *EMBO Reports. Science and Society* 3 (8), 703–706.
Whitley, R. (1985) Knowledge producers and knowledge acquirers: Popularisation as a relation between scientific fields and their publics. In T. Shinn and R. Whitley (eds) *Expository Science: Forms and Functions of Popularization* (pp. 3–28). Dordrecht: Reidel.
Widdowson, H.G. (1979) *Explorations in Applied Linguistics*. Oxford: Oxford University Press.

Appendix 1

A sample of Corpus A (RAs) corresponding to *The Lancet* journal (front page).

The Lancet
Lancet 2001; 358 (9285): 903-911
September 15, 2001

Rheumatoid **arthritis**

SOURCE: Division of Rheumatology, Department of Medicine, Brigham and Women's Hospital, 75 Francis Street, Boston, MA 02115, USA (D M Lee MD, M E Weinblatt MD)

Correspondence to: Dr Michael E Weinblatt (e-mail: mweinblatt@partners.org)

AUTHOR: David M Lee, Michael E Weinblatt

SECTION: Review

LENGTH: 6444 words

Rheumatoid **arthritis** is a systemic inflammatory disorder that mainly affects the diarthrodial joint. It is the most common form of inflammatory **arthritis,** and has a substantial societal effect in terms of cost, disability, and lost productivity. Although the pathogenesis of rheumatoid **arthritis** remains incompletely understood, much insight into the cellular and molecular mechanisms involved has been gained in the past decade. On the basis of these insights, new therapies have been developed, and clinical trials have shown the efficacy of aggressive treatment of patients with active disease. In this review, we discuss improvements in our understanding of the pathophysiology of inflammatory synovitis in rheumatoid **arthritis,** and improvements in therapy for patients with the disorder. The past decade has seen substantial advances in these areas. Future studies will be directed at improving methods for early diagnosis and identification of patients with progressive disease, and at improving methods to identify candidates for subclasses of disease-modifying antirheumatic drugs (DMARDs). Long-term safety and efficacy data for the new DMARD agents and combination regimens will also further delineate efficacy and toxicity and thus the appropriate clinical context for use of these therapeutic approaches. The continuing elucidation of pathophysiological pathways relevant in rheumatoid **arthritis,** coupled with continuing advances in biotechnology and rational drug design, offer substantial hope for the continued development of increasingly potent and specific pharmacotherapy for treatment of rheumatoid **arthritis.**

Rheumatoid **arthritis** affects about 1% of the population, in a female/male ratio of 2.5/1. The disease can occur at any age, but it is most common among those aged 40-70 years, its incidence increasing with age. The geographic distribution of rheumatoid **arthritis** is worldwide, with a notably low prevalence in rural Africa and high prevalence in specific tribes of Native Americans (Pima and Chippewa). There is no clear association between prevalence of rheumatoid **arthritis** and socioeconomic status.

Clinical features

The range of presentations of rheumatoid **arthritis** is broad, but disease onset is insidious in most cases, and several months can elapse before a firm diagnosis can be ascertained. The predominant symptoms are pain, stiffness, and swelling of peripheral joints (panel 1).

Appendix 2

A sample of Corpus B (AR4) corresponding to *Science Daily* website (front page).

Featured Research

from universities, journals, and other organizations

Hip replacement an excellent option for young juvenile arthritis patients

Date: November 17, 2014

Source: Hospital for Special Surgery

Summary: Total hip replacement is an excellent option for patients under age 35 when conservative treatments fail to provide pain relief, researchers have found. The implant lasted at least 10 years in 85 percent of patients.

Share This

Email to a friend

- Facebook
- Twitter
- LinkedIn
- Google +
- Print this page

When you think of hip replacement surgery, you generally envision an older adult with painful osteoarthritis. But the procedure is also used for younger patients with juvenile idiopathic arthritis (JIA) whose joints have been severely damaged by the disease.

Related Articles

- Anesthesia
- Sleep disorder
- Opioid drug

- MMR vaccine
- Delirium
- Chronic pain

A new study by Hospital for Special Surgery (HSS) researchers finds that total hip replacement (THR) is an excellent option for patients under age 35 when conservative treatments fail to provide relief.

The study, presented at the American College of Rheumatology annual meeting on November 16, found that hip replacement lasted at least 10 years in 85 percent of JIA patients. Twenty years out, 50 percent of the patients needed a revision surgery, or second hip replacement.

Juvenile idiopathic arthritis is a common rheumatologic disease in children that often persists into adulthood. It frequently affects the hip joint, and total hip replacement is the standard treatment to relieve pain and restore mobility when nonsurgical treatments no longer help.

'The surgery in this patient population, although performed by only a small number of specialized orthopedic surgeons nationwide, is life-changing for JIA patients,' said Mark P. Figgie, M.D., senior author of the study and chief of the Surgical Arthritis Service at HSS. 'Joint replacement can free patients from a life of unrelenting pain. It can enable those in a wheel chair to walk again. Patients can go back to school or work and get their lives back.'

5 The Ethics of Informed Consent. An Applied Linguistics Perspective

Morten Pilegaard

As healthcare becomes a major factor in the national and global economy, a wide range of ethical challenges emerge. Although relevant to all human and communicative behaviour, ethics is particularly important in communication about health because it brings to light special concerns related to life and death and to mental and physical well-being that are rarely as significant in other contexts. Ethical concerns are inherent in nearly every kind of health communication (HC). The present chapter explores the issue of ethics in informed consent documents (ICDs) from an applied linguistics (AL) perspective and suggests a framework for analysing how dimensions of ethicalness surface linguistically in ICDs. Specifically, the study seeks to (a) inform the ongoing discussion of the ethics of informed consent (IC), offering insights obtained by using AL and by drawing parallels with relevant findings obtained from the study of other HC genres; (b) suggest a multidisciplinary AL approach to the study of ICDs that broadens the perspective on ethicalness to comprise text structure and rhetorical functions, and that takes the description of the issue of comprehension problems to a deeper level of semantic categories and lexico-grammar; and (c) apply this framework in an analysis of a sample of Danish ICDs.

Background

Health communication

As healthcare becomes a major factor in the national and global economy, a wide range of ethical challenges emerge. Although relevant to all human and communicative behaviour, ethics is particularly important in communication about health (henceforth health communication [HC]) because it brings to light special concerns related to life and death and to mental and physical well-being that are rarely as significant in other contexts. Ethical concerns are inherent in nearly every kind of HC, including how communication should be framed and what patients should or should not be told. The present chapter's focus on ethics and language is mirrored in the growing recognition of the need to tailor communication to specific patient groups' knowledge levels, the growing awareness of patients' and citizens' diverse health information-seeking behaviour (Anker *et al.*, 2011) and the growing focus on patient empowerment and joint decision-making (Chewning *et al.*, 2012). This chapter responds to the need for insights into how ethics translates into communication to obtain informed consent (IC) to participate in medical research, which is a pertinent issue (Treweek *et al.*, 2013).

Ethics in healthcare

Various influential applied ethical paradigms may be identified in HC. Utilitarianism argues that ethical decisions should be taken in accordance with the greatest happiness (or welfare) of the greatest number of people. The use of cost–benefit or cost–utility analyses is a current example of utilitarianism. Becoming ever more pervasive in health economists', hospital administrators' and policymakers' discourse, the utilitarian approach shows in coinages like 'health technology assessment' and 'quality-adjusted life years', to mention a few. In this approach, ethics justifies itself on the basis of the net economic benefit of a healthcare initiative to society regardless of its impact on individuals' rights.

Virtue ethics focuses on individuals' moral behaviour and has been applied to the interpersonal context, where healthcare providers are expected to be virtuous and guided by their commitment to do what is right. For example, bioethics offers clinicians salient theories or models to resolve diagnostic dilemmas. But 'while medicine is characterised by objective "truth", ethical discourse is not amenable to such "truths"' (Danbury *et al.*, 2010: 6). The professional can therefore find no 'truths' in these models about what and how to tell the patient. In this approach, ethics is concerned with how communication reflects particular, personal qualities like honesty, integrity, courage and compassion in the dispositions and responses (Radden & Sadler, 2010).

In Kantian deontology, the starting point is the individual's inherent worth. Central to this approach is Kant's categorical imperative, which rests on the idea that one should never treat people as a mere means to an end, and that an individual's worth lies in that individual's ability as a rational being to direct his or her own life. This chapter adopts Kant's deontology. First, it makes sense both as a fundamental ethical doctrine and as applied to our specific area, where the *individual* has to give IC. Second, Kantian ethics underpins existing understandings of IC, according to Vaughn (2010: 216): 'The heart of the modern doctrine of IC is Kantian. Because persons are autonomous, rational agents, they must be allowed the freedom to make choices and to have them respected'. The Kantian principle of respect is encoded in national and international guidelines on IC, which require that information must be provided, that the information is comprehensible and that consent to participate is given voluntarily (WHO, 2012). IC therefore not only describes a process whereby an individual's voluntary approval to participation is given after the purpose of the study, its risks and alternatives have been described thoroughly both orally and in writing. IC is also deeply concerned with communication, the way communication takes place and the context in which it unfolds, because obtaining IC is a purposeful attempt to influence personal behaviour.

Informed consent in bioethics research

Extant bioethics literature has investigated the issue of IC in the context of medical research, and the literature is unanimous that IC is not sufficiently ethical because participants in medical experiments often find it difficult to understand the documents on which consent rests (IC documents [ICDs]) (Pandiya, 2010; Schenker *et al.*, 201; Terranova *et al.*, 2012) and therefore cannot consent on an informed basis. Many studies have evaluated research participants' ability to understand ICDs by using quantitative measurements of lexical and syntactical complexity based on, for instance, the number of letters per word and the number of words and syllables per sentence (e.g. the Flesch reading ease score [Flesch, 1948], the Gunning Fog Index [Gunning, 1952] and the Fry scale [Fry, 1968]).

Readability formulas, however, are 'imperfect predictors of text readability and understandability or comprehension' (Zamanian & Heydari, 2012: 47). First, they largely ignore situational or contextual parameters, which lie at the heart of any act of communication, and any rendering of the consent process that fails to recognise the social and cultural construction of IC as an act of communication falls short of adequacy. Second, the process of providing information and obtaining consent takes place within the context of a conversation between a healthcare professional and a potential participant in that research. This process is essentially dialogical and must (Marta, 1996) take into account the linguistic complexity of the act of communication, the fact that the act of giving consent follows after a series of speech acts that together form a polyphonic, heteroglossial discourse presenting many, potentially conflicting, perspectives. Third, because readability formulas are composed of the variables of words and sentence length, they characterise the surface structure of a text, not its deeper syntactic and semantic structures. Fourth, they do not consider the overall structure or organisation of the text. Traditionally, monodisciplinary bioethics studies using readability as a proxy for ethicalness therefore fail to capture important ethical dimensions of communication related to the IC process and its texts.

Various models for understanding the IC process exist (e.g. Faden & Beauchamps, 1986), but they do not account for the linguistic underpinnings of IC and therefore fail to identify the factors that obscure, prevent or jeopardise communication in the IC process. It is almost as if language is assumed to be a non-factor in itself (Marta, 1996). Failing to appreciate the social, contextual and, indeed, cultural construction of IC as an act of communication (Appelbaum *et al.*, 1987), the traditional medico-legal model of IC sees communication as a 'disclosure process', i.e. a linear series of acts of communication where the participants have clearly defined roles. Following Marta (1996: 42) 'the physician discloses information, the patient understands, and a decision is made. Here disclosure and comprehension are juxtaposed but distinct and discontinuous. The physician is an informer only, the patient a consenter or refuser only'.

Informed consent in linguistics

Marta (1996: 56) criticises this disclosure model and proposes a model for linguistic analysis of the IC process based on language philosophy, structural linguistics and literary analysis in which IC is conceived as a performative speech act in the sense that it elicits a verbal act (i.e. that of granting or refusing consent) after a conversation has taken place in which 'distinct individuals, multiple voices, and multiple perspectives have been respected, and convention observed and recognized'. Marta's (1996: 44) model neatly captures the socially construed complexity of the IC process and its integration with Kantian ethics by reinforcing 'the adherence of informed consent to its underlying ethical rationale of respect for persons'. However, it fails to get much closer to identifying *how* ethics surface in the actual language used.

We therefore need a more holistic, interdisciplinary approach focused on language. This chapter seeks to make a contribution to the field of applied bioethics. It focuses on ICDs and proposes a model for how various applied linguistics (AL) disciplines may offer insights into where the problems of 'unethicalness' lie. It builds partly on the systemic functional linguistics (SFL) framework proposed by Clerehan *et al.* (2005), yet supplements this by suggesting how other AL theories may enrich our understanding of ICDs' ethicalness.

Rationale and aim

The AL approach is chosen because the chapter's concern is with the practical issue of how ethics are discursively constructed in 'real-world' texts. The AL approach invites inclusion of issues relevant to the text as well as the context (see 'Design').

While the use of AL is not alien to the study of the process of obtaining IC in face-to-face verbal encounters (e.g. Ness *et al.*, 2009), to our knowledge only three recent studies (Pilegaard & Ravn, 2012, 2013; Sand *et al.*, 2012) have so far approached the issue of 'ethicalness' in ICDs. These three studies confirm the findings of previous bioethics studies (e.g. Terblanche & Burgess, 2011), namely that the understanding of the ICDs is hampered, e.g. due to lexical density and the use of specialised terminology to designate core concepts.

The purpose of this chapter is to explore the issue of ethics in ICDs from an AL perspective and to suggest a framework for analysing how dimensions of ethicalness surface linguistically in ICDs.

Many non-linguistic issues with a potential bearing on the ethicalness of ICDs as defined here are ignored for reasons of space, e.g. graphical presentation like length, format, layout and use of visuals – and, for example, the use of headlines indicating macro themes (Martin, 1992).

Theory

Patient centredness

Patient centredness (PC) occupies a key position in modern healthcare. Its philosophy is that the healthcare provider understands the patient as a person, not as a cluster of diseases (Epstein, 2000). The assumed values are that patients are qualified to decide their own needs and expectations, and that they can make decisions and choices about what they need and want (Lutz & Bowers, 2000). Coulter (2002) defines PC communication as 'Health care that meets and responds to patients' wants, needs and preferences and where patients are autonomous and able to decide for themselves'. In PC theory, patients are unique individuals whose needs, preferences and values are respected and catered for during interaction. This value is so fundamental that it outranks other interests as illustrated in the Danish Act on Research Ethics Review of Health Research Projects: 'Consideration for the rights, safety and well-being of trial subjects come before scientific and social interests in the possibilities of gaining new knowledge or investigating existing knowledge that may justify the undertaking of a research project' (Den Nationale Videnskabsetiske Komité, 2014).

The PC paradigm focuses on doctor–patient interaction in the clinical setting, and it is rarely mentioned in the IC ethics literature. A review of randomised control trials (RCTs) (Edwards *et al.*, 1998) reported no mention of PC in any of the 812 papers reviewed. Even so, the ethical importance of PC shows in professional codes, guidelines and standards wherein core ethical principles form a comprehensive, consensus-based ethical framework for how to care for any person in a situation of vulnerability. This implicit reference to PC relies on principalism, which establishes an ethical basis for action based on specific rules or principles (e.g. autonomy, beneficence and justice) as reflected in Section 26 of the World Medical Association's rendition of the Declaration of Helsinki (WMA, 2013): 'Special attention should be given to the specific information needs of individual potential subjects as well as to the methods used to deliver the information'. But principalism is just one approach to moral philosophy. Other ethical and philosophical movements and methods provide additional ethical bases for patient-centred communication.

Owing to Immanuel Kant, most deontological ethical theories hold that all humans are morally required to respect the autonomy of other persons. A key issue concerning patient-centred communication is the relationship between patient-centred communication and autonomy: If patient-centred communication is sensitive to autonomy, then it is a moral good.

In the context of IC, PC has been associated with the clinical situation, including that where consent is sought; yet little has been achieved in terms of tailoring written information to individual patients' needs (Bridson *et al.*, 2003). Still, many PC core values can successfully be extended to text as discussed by Fage-Butler (2013) for patient package inserts (PPIs).

Comprehension

The ethical imperative of IC implies that lay friendliness (LF) is a key feature of the ICD. According to Vaughn (2010: 9), it is ethically problematic if patients do not understand IC forms, as 'choices cannot be considered entirely autonomous unless they are fully informed'. Still, we side with recent critique of the bioethics/principalist approach, e.g. as voiced by the British philosopher Onora O'Neill (Manson & O'Neill, 2011), who argues that being fully informed is rarely achievable in practice. Along with Nisbeth Jensen (2013), we therefore take a pragmatic approach both to the concept of LF, which is conceptualised as the simple legal requirement that IDSs must be easy to understand; and to the concept of PC, which is conceptualised in accordance with Section B, Article 24 of the World Medical Association, viz. that 'special attention should be given to the specific information needs of individual potential subjects as well as to the methods used to deliver the information'. This special attention to the individual's information *needs* and his or her *ability* to understand what is being communicated lies at the core of Kantian deontology. In this chapter, ethicalness is accordingly conceptualised as lay friendliness/patient centredness (LFPC).

By using the term LF rather than readability, we avoid the simplified view of text comprehension reflected in the traditional biomedical mechanistic, transmissionist one-way communication models (Nisbeth Jensen, 2013). We also divorce ourselves from the view that a text's quality can be assessed simply by studying the document itself. The concept of LF has been successfully applied in various linguistic and translational approaches to other mandatory genres such as PPIs (e.g. Nisbeth Jensen, 2013). It has only recently been employed in a study of ICDs (Pilegaard &

Ravn, 2013), which showed that ICDs are generally not lay friendly because they are difficult to understand for lay people.

The issue of comprehension is closely related to that of health literacy defined as 'the cognitive and social skills determining the motivation and ability of people to gain access to, understand, and use information in ways that promote and maintain good health' (WHO, 1998: 10). In this definition, health literacy is more than just the ability to read and understand (i.e. 'functional' literacy); it also includes 'conceptual' literacy, which has been defined as 'a multi-dimensional approach that links generic skills with a body of technical and cultural knowledge that give meaning to the skills, and situates the individual in a social context', i.e. the individual's ability to make informed choices (Kanj & Mitic, 2009: 14). This definition responds to the call for a definition that goes beyond comprehension of the written word and patients' interaction with the healthcare system (e.g. Kickbusch, 2001), and it acknowledges the importance of the social context. General measures of health literacy like the REALM, the TOFHLA and Newest Vital Sign test instruments (Kajn & Mitic, 2009) mainly test reading proficiency and cannot be used for assessing health literacy as defined here, and they will therefore not be discussed.

Text and context

The ICD is inherently value laden and involves many, occasionally conflicting, interests. ICDs are therefore fraught with ethical peril when addressing issues like benefit and risk. These issues must be carefully and ethically handled, and any such handling is subject to the dynamics of the context in which they unfold. A key premise here is therefore that ethicalness is contextual in the sense that it arises from an interaction between the context, the text and its reader. Following this line of argument, we must study the context to understand the texts, we must study the texts to understand the language and we must study the language to unveil how ethicalness is discursively constructed in ICDs. This line of reasoning, albeit in the reverse order, has been voiced before (Halliday & Hasan, 1989), but to the author's knowledge, only a few studies have sought to apply this insight in an interdisciplinary AL approach to the study of HC, and none have so far investigated ICDs in this way.

Design

Interdiscipline

As context and communication may be analysed individually but cannot be comprehended separately, we must focus on a variety of analytical variables like how the context shapes the text; the amount, structure and relevance of the information provided; the clarity, intelligibility and comprehensibility of the language used; the attention given to the involved parties' needs and abilities; and the speech acts involved in granting consent. This variety of analytical dimensions commands an interdisciplinary applied linguistics (AP) approach to capture the full breadth of this text–context–agent interplay. We here use genre analysis, register and lexis analysis, discourse analysis and translation analysis to inform the bioethics discussion of ethicalness, i.e. lay-friendliness/patient-centeredness (LFPC), in the ICD.

Genre

The ICD is an institutionally, socially recognised way of using language (Hyland, 2002) to achieve a particular objective. We use genre theory to understand the social construction of the ICD as a text. This chapter positions itself between two approaches to genre theory. In the new rhetoric approach, drawing on Berkenkotter and Huckin (1995), genre is seen as 'the motivated, functional relationship between text type and rhetorical situation' (Coe *et al.*, 2002: 195). This tradition tends to be ethnographic rather than text analytic. The other main approach stresses the social purposes of genres and the schematic structures serving these purposes. In this tradition, genre is a goal-oriented approach (Martin, 1992), and the ways in which language is used are linked systematically to the context of culture and the context of situation. The methodologies tend to explain the rhetorical structure of genres and the patterns of grammatical, cohesive and lexical choices (Christie & Martin, 1997; Martin, 1997) inspired by SFL. This chapter occupies a middle ground by employing Bhatia's approach to the interdiscursive mediation of ICDs, i.e. the ICDs' recognisable structural identity arises in response to contextual demands and the genre's goal-directedness, and it argues that genre theory mainly contributes to explain the ICD's rhetorical structure.

The ICD is a mandated genre, heavily regulated by international institutions (European Parliament, 2001; WHO, 2013) and national agencies, e.g. the UK Medicines for Human Use Regulation (National Health Service, 2015). It has a set information structure that can be interpreted as functional parts of text, called *moves* and *steps*. This approach was successfully used to describe the specific macro- (move) and micro- (step) levels of rhetorical structure in Danish ICDs (Pilegaard & Ravn, 2013) with each step having a particular rhetorical sub-function, viz. to inform, to instruct, etc., subsumed under the superordinate function of achieving IC.

Genre analysis may help break down the text into functional units of variable length, and we suggest that ethicalness springs from the order of these moves and steps and from their verbal realisation. In ICDs, some moves, like that of informing the reader about the voluntariness of participation, may be seen as more essential than others, and they should therefore be placed first. In the analysis, we focus on these first moves.

Permission to conduct research with human test subjects is granted by regional research ethics committees (RECs) on the basis, among others, of the patient information sheet (PIS) and the consent form, which together constitute the ICDs. An REC may request changes in the PIS or reject the application if it is deemed to pose comprehension problems. An REC's approval of a project is not just a neutral administrative act; it is also an explicit endorsement of the project's ethical qualities, i.e. its LFPC. Although the approval procedure could be analysed purely in terms of protection from ethical issues related to problematic research, the presence of lay members on most RECs suggests another possible function, namely that of guaranteeing that the information given to prospective research participants is lay friendly/patient centred. On this minimal interpretation, the lay persons' role on the REC board is that of a linguistic sounding board (Pilegaard & Ravn, 2012).

The literature on lay REC members' evaluation of the comprehensibility of ICDs is scarce. Yet, a large UK National Health Service (NHS) study of lay REC members (Simons *et al.*, 2009: 15) reported that 'the main barrier identified by respondents to full participation in RECs was the language used by the applicants in their lay summaries as well as in their full applications'. We are apparently facing the paradox that although international and national guidelines offer directions as to the structure of ICDs and some concrete advice to enhance LFPC, the reality of the language used in PIS apparently resists this advice. In the words of the NHS (2011: 90) itself, 'There is evidence that improvement is possible'. To get one step closer to understanding why this is so, we use register analysis to explore the actual language used.

Register analysis

Register analysis is concerned with language variation (e.g. Halliday, 1978; Halliday & Hassan, 1989) and sees register as a functionally defined language variety; hence, the particular contextual configuration in which a given communicative event takes place is expressed through the selection of certain types of meaning to the exclusion of others. Where genre is concerned with the contextual determinants of realisable rhetorical structures, register analysis is concerned with how context impacts on the verbal instantiation of these structures. We may illustrate this using the tripartite configuration of contextual factors (field, tenor and mode) proposed by Eggins (1994).

Briefly, the concept of field, an element of the cognitive or experiential metafunction of a text, captures both the social activity in which the communicants are engaged and what is commonly referred to as the subject matter. For simplicity, we here consider field only as the lexical items describing the subject matter and will not discuss other elements of register like process and circumstance. The concept of tenor, a component of the interpersonal metafunction of a text, is the social relation between the interactants in the communicative situation. In Eggins's (1994: 100) use of SFL, tenor is conceptualised into levels of formality that spring from the variables power, contact and affective involvement. In the IC situation, the context is characterised by unequal power, rare contact and little emotional involvement, and formality will accordingly tend to be high. Mode is an element of textual metafunction. A text can be modelled as a point in a continuum defined by axes such as spoken/written and action/reflection oriented. The concept of mode is the most 'opaque part of Halliday and Hasan's definition of context' (Hill-Madsen, 2014: 31). Mode will therefore here be used only in the sense of 'medium' (Halliday & Hasan, 1989) spanning from spoken to written. We consider only the traditional, paper-based medium, as the use of other media seems not to 'significantly improve knowledge of consent information' (Agre *et al.*, 2003: 17).

Hill-Madsen (2014: 268–269) identifies seven principles ordered along clines of lay orientedness of relevance for the fulfilment of the PIS's function – or *skopos* (Vermeer, 1996) – of being LF. The principle most unequivocally contributing to enhance accessibility is neutralisation which involves shifts between alternative lexico-grammatical instantiations like decrease in technicality, decrease in formality, non-technical paraphrase, informal paraphrase, shift in theme from marked to unmarked, shift in voice from receptive to operative, etc. Among these, especially, a decrease in technicality and non-technical paraphrase seem absolute prerequisites for the fulfilment of the lay-oriented skopos, according to Hill-Madsen (2014).

Register analysis may help us understand how context shapes the choice of lexico-grammatical instantiations and may help us navigate along clines of lay centredness at multiple and highly granulated levels to fulfil the PIS's ethical skopos.

Translation analysis

Register analysis provides a tool for analysing the lexico-grammatical instantiations of verbal meaning, but does not explain why the register of the ICDs leans towards the expert rather than the lay spectrum. To understand why this is so, we may look to translation analysis; here, broadly conceived also as intra-lingual translation, i.e. an interpretation of verbal signs by means of other signs of the same language (Jakobson, 1959/2000; Zethsen, 2007, 2009). In this view, a medical expert producing a PIS for a lay reader may be conceived of as a translator performing intra-lingual translation or rewording of a text in a different style within the same language. The literature on intra-lingual rewording/translation in HC is almost non-existent. Still, Muñoz-Miquel (2012) identifies a number of macro-textual and micro-textual or lexico-grammatical changes (e.g. sentence length and structure, verbs and voice, noun phrases, tenor and modality) that take place to ease comprehension in the production of lay summaries from medical research papers. Furthermore, a study by Ezpeleta-Piorno (2012) on the rewriting or intra-lingual translation processes when PPIs are produced on the basis of a summary of product characteristics (SPCs) notes that 'readability appears to be related mainly to a decrease in technicality (field) and possibly to a lessening of the written character of the texts (mode) and the enhancement of personalisation is related to a decrease in formality (tenor)' (quoted in Hill-Madsen, 2014: 77).

In the intra-lingual translation literature (e.g. Askehave & Zethsen, 2003), it is recommended to use the lowest common denominator approach in intra-language translation of functional texts intended for a lay reader. Working from this, Nisbeth Jensen argues that plain language as a concept can be viewed as a type of intra-lingual translation, because its aim is to *translate* a complex monolingual text into a plainer and more easily read and understood lay text (Nisbeth Jensen, 2015: 169). Based on a review of the literature, she proposes a 'comprehensibility framework' of generally agreed elements that should be avoided because they represent 'consensus in the literature concerning that which makes a text difficult or easy to understand linguistically at the word and sentence levels' (Nisbeth Jensen, 2015: 171).

Translation analysis may help determine how translational remnants (interlingual/ intra-lingual) detrimental to LF may be traced and to which extent such expert tenor and mode remnants may be further reworded/ translated into lay tenor.

Discourse analysis

IC involves communication through the use of language, and language is a powerful mechanism for social control (Fairclough, 1992). In relation to the ethics dimension of ICDs and the obligation not to coerce, deceive or manipulate (see 'Comprehension'), we may examine how ethicalness is discursively constructed and how power relations unfold discursively in ICDs. For this purpose, we may supplement the above linguistically oriented approaches with Foucauldian discourse analytic (FDA). FDA offers insight into the underlying assumptions textually constructing the sender, the receiver and the contents of the ICD – elements that are critical to the ethicalness of ICDs.

FDA has been used to examine oral negotiations about IC but not the ethical aspects in ICDs. Yet, in a paper aiming to find means for evaluating PPIs sensitive to patients' complaints, Fage-Butler (2013) uses FDA to analyse discursive statements in texts. Having identified statements, Fage-Butler (2012: 10) formulates questions to identify their underlying functions focused on PC. The statements relate to the construction of the sender and help disclose the ethical stance (e.g. is the sender's expertise balanced with acknowledgement of the patient's knowledge?), the main discursive content (e.g. do discourses reflect an interest in the patient as a person?) and – importantly for the present purpose – the receiver (e.g. is the receiver characterised as a unique individual?). Fage-Butler demonstrates that in many statements, PC is minimal or entirely absent, and that when the patient is constructed discursively, the biomedical construction is dominant.

Discourse analysis may help us identify both the explicit and implicit assumptions in the discursive construction of the interactants.

Linguistic frameworks for analysis of HC genres

In the search for how LFPC is discursively constructed, we may draw on an evaluative linguistic framework (ELF) for analysis of patient information leaflets (PILs) (Clerehan *et al*., 2005).Using the ELF, Hirsh *et al*. (2009) conclude that leaflets generated from a linguistic framework are clearer and more effective in communicating information about medications. The ELF has also been found useful for ICD analysis (Sand & Eik-Nes, 2012). This study reported a change in the relative 'functional readability' of Norwegian ICDs over time. The conclusions were based on consideration of the following items, for each of which 'readability' was defined partly based on ELF as shown in parentheses: (1) generic structure (readability equivalent to reader's expectations concerning content being met), (2) rhetorical functions (readability equivalent to reader knowing what to do with text), (3) reader–writer relationship (readability equivalent to reader being able to identify actors and relationships between them and these elements being consistently and adequately presented), (4) meta-discourse (readability equivalent to reader having verbal clues signalling what he/she is supposed to do with the information), (5) headings (readability equivalent to reader getting an impression of the main themes and how they are related), (6) technicality of vocabulary (readability equivalent to reader being familiar with the terminology and use of lay terms) and (7) visual aspects (readability equivalent to reader being helped to navigate the document using visual aspects like illustrations, typographical clues, etc.). These definitions clearly resonate with the LFPC stance taken in this chapter.

Methods and Materials

Materials

The material consists of 10 randomly chosen PISs from 258 ICDs submitted to the Central Denmark and Capital Region RECs in Denmark for approval during 2008–2009. Text samples are drawn purposefully only from the first two moves of these PISs, and the samples are translated into English to illustrate how the AL disciplines may be applied to trace LFPC.

Methods

The AL analytical lenses are applied consecutively and operationalised through a number of key questions. Using the lens of genre theory, the LFPC of the PIS may be examined based on questions exploring the structure of the text: Does the move and step structure clearly reflect the purpose of the text? Is the main rhetorical purpose established early in the text as a frame? Using the SFL lens of register analysis, LFPC may be determined from answers to these questions: Can the lexical items be deemed comprehensible to the lay reader? Is the relationship between sender and receiver clear, and is the reader recognised as a unique individual? Exploring LFPC through the lens of translation analysis, we may ask whether the PIS contains lexical and lexico-grammatical instances or remnants of expert register and mode. Does the text contain elements detrimental to LFPC, such as specialised terminology, officialese, nominalisations, passives, compounds and synonyms? Can anything be simplified? Investigating the LFPC using discourse analysis, the following question may be asked: Are statements about sender, receiver and contents discursively constructed in an ethical way, i.e. with a focus on the receiver characterised as a unique individual with a lived, valuable experience of concern to the sender?

Findings and Discussion

Genre analysis

Examining the first two moves (introduction and purpose) and their constituent steps, eight PISs had the recommended PIS move order. These eight PISs also requested participation as the first step of the first move. In the remaining two PISs, participation was requested at the end of the introduction move. None used headlines specifically denoting the rhetorical function (request). Most text samples failed to include all the recommended steps in the introduction move, viz. (1) 'Request participation'; (2) 'Refer to annexed informed consent form and consent certificate'; (3) 'Explain why you are inviting the subject to participate'; (4) 'State who you are and who took the research initiative'; (5) 'Invite subject to carefully read the PIS and assure the subject that participation is entirely voluntary'.

This order of steps is meant to leave the reader in no doubt about the text's purpose from its very beginning, which is tantamount to ethicalness at the structural level. Failure to clearly signal this purpose early on reduces a text's ethicalness. In line with Sand and Eik-Nes (2012), we claim that the text should be oriented towards the trial participant as the main reader, and this can be achieved by textually fronting the step in which consent is requested. We speculate (Pilegaard & Ravn, 2012) that some of the steps in the introduction move are left out because PIS authors find that inclusion of too much information in the PIS detracts from its readability, as also noted by Sand and Eik-Nes (2012: 67). Yet we find it problematic that the structural elements left out are those that pertain to the ethical skopos of the PIS.

In conclusion, contextual constraints seem detrimental to LFPC. First, practice defies recommendations on the number, order and contents of steps in the first moves of the PIS, presumably because these recommendations are seen by the discourse community as being at odds with 'the rationale which shapes the schematic structure and constrains the choice of content and style' (Swales, 1990: 58). Defying these recommendations is tantamount to 'structural unethicalness'.

Register analysis

Field

The goal of reading is to derive meaning. Yet titles and the first two moves revealed many unexplained, lexical nouns designating descriptive and topographic anatomy, physiology, diagnostic procedures and medicines from which the lay reader may derive little meaning. In three cases, the titles framing the IC were lay oriented (e.g. 'The functioning of the anus in people with spinal cord injury'). Six titles effectively barred lay comprehension, e.g. 'Urinary aquaporin excretion pre- and post-TIPS therapy in cirrhotic patients with portal hypertension' and 'Effect of thoracoscopic sympadectomy on cardiopulmonary function assessed from pulse variability and CPX'. From an ethical perspective focusing on field, this is deemed unethical.

All PISs contained lexical items that were deemed difficult to comprehend for the intended reader. Especially problematic was the use of technical words in the introduction move's third step ('Explain why you are inviting the subject to participate') and in the first step ('Explain the purpose of the experiment') of the purpose move. These steps are essential because if neither the overall nor the specific purpose is clear, the whole basis of the IC is unethical because it is uninformed. These two steps contained many not adequately 'neutralised' (Hill-Madsen, 2014) items. An example: 'The purpose of this trial is to compare the effect (positive as well as negative) of treatment with parathyroid hormone (PTH (1-48) with alendronate on lumbar pain due to cervical collapse'. Here, a short and non-technical explanation of 'parathyroid hormone' and 'alendronate' could have reduced the technicality. Still, the PISs also contained many examples of 'neutralised' lexical items, e.g. 'The purpose of this experiment is to examine if a new method (micro dialysis) can be used to describe the regulation of the blood flow in healthy adults'. Here, the non-technical term ('new method') is used and the technical word is in brackets ('micro dialysis').

Inconsistency characterised the level of technicality of the lexical items within and across the PISs examined. Some PISs contained many unexplained 'content' words and were overall 'lexically dense' (Clerehan *et al.*, 2004: 338). Others tended to be 'lexically dense' only occasionally, typically in moves explaining procedures. The choice of lexical items was thus not consistently guided by consideration for the intended readers' level of understanding and familiarity with the terms used.

We speculate that a tension exists between the mandatory use of lay language and a deeply embedded expert language practice among PIS producers. The collegial practice of allegiance with the expert domain, confidence in using the expert register and a propensity to favour the formal, precise register of science over the less precise lay language is likely to incline PIS producers towards the expert field, while knowing that the PIS must be understandable to the intended reader to receive REC approval. We also speculate that a PIS producer may well wish to put a low processing load on the reader through low lexical density, yet may be unable linguistically to navigate along clines of lay orientedness for want of linguistic insight as previously noted (Pilegaard, 2006).

Tenor

Analysis of tenor in moves 1 and 2 showed that the reader was referred to either directly as a patient in the introduction move Step 1 ('Request participation') about to undergo treatment, e.g. 'As you are a patient scheduled for haemodialysis, we would like to ask you…' or indirectly as a member of a group of readers ('We are inviting 20 patients and 20 healthy volunteers in order to investigate...'). Group reference was more prevalent than patient reference in Step 3 ('Explain why you are inviting the subject to participate'). Interestingly, seven PISs were reader oriented rather than sender based, mentioning the reader before the writer. In three cases, Step 1 ('Request participation') of move 1 was formulated 'bald-on-record' (Brown & Levinson, 1987), (e.g. 'You are hereby requested to participate in…'), i.e. without redressive face-work to mitigate the illocutionary force of the request; in other cases, politeness markers were used (e.g. 'You are hereby kindly requested to participate in…').

Three cases were sender based, opening Step 1 ('Request participation') of move 1 (introduction) with sentences like 'We would like to ask you whether you want to…' or 'I hereby ask you if you will participate in…'. However, only two PISs identified the sender's name, role and departmental affiliation as recommended (Step 4, 'State who you are and who took the research initiative'), e.g. 'The project's principal investigator is ... based at ... hospital'; two PISs failed to identify the sender at all.

Failure to identify the sender and to assign clear roles to the interactants is evidence of poor LFPC at the level of tenor; this is particularly so if the reader is described as an object of investigation rather than as a unique individual, and failure to redress the face-threatening act of requesting linguistically deprives the potential participant of freedom of choice.

In the Norwegian ICDs, readers were addressed personally as 'you' and in the third person either as a member of a whole group of readers or as possible members of a subgroup of readers. The two forms were frequently used within the same document (Sand & Eik-Nes, 2012: 72), but no account was given as to how readers were addressed in particular moves or steps, even if this may be especially interesting from an ethical point of view. We argue that addressing the reader using a personal pronoun early in the text is tantamount to ethicalness at the level of tenor.

Translation analysis

As seen in 'Register analysis', specialised terminology abounded in titles and first moves, among others in Step 1 ('Request participation', introduction), e.g. 'As you are a patient scheduled for haemodialysis...' and 'You are hereby requested to participate in a scientific experiment concerning the excretion of urinary aquaporins pre and post TIPS therapy in cirrhotic patients with portal hypertension'. The first example contains the Latin-based expert term 'haemodialysis', presumably because no Danish lay term exists; yet, the meaning could have been explained, e.g. 'the removal of fluid and waste products from the blood' to ease comprehension. Likewise, the English abbreviation 'TRIPS' (transjugular intrahepatic portosystemic shunt) exemplifies both interlingual and intra-lingual translation 'failure'. In the other example, the Latin-based word 'cirrhotic' instead of the fully equivalent Danish lay word 'skrumpelever' illustrates the failure of intra-lingual translation from the expert's to the layperson's register. We presume that medical professionals may often not appreciate the large difference between lay and expert medical terminology in Danish unlike English (Pilegaard, 1997a) or see no need to render the concept in lay language because of the extensive use of Latin- and Greek-based words in Danish language, not generally but in expert HC (Pilegaard, 2006: 171).

The most notable example of *officialese*, i.e. formal and overly complex prose belonging to the official register, is found in a phrase repeatedly used in Step 1, 'You are hereby requested to participate in...'). The use of officialese ('hereby' and the formal word 'requested' rather than 'asked') combined with the passive ('requested') rather than the active voice adds to the formality of the PIS and introduces a distance counterproductive to LFPC. In the two moves examined, though, most of the PISs use less formal and less official expressions, e.g. 'I would like to ask you if you want to participate in...'.

The PISs contained a large number of nominalisations, especially in Move 2 'Purpose' (Step 1, 'State general purpose'), e.g. 'The purpose of this trial is to investigate the likelihood of patients with carpal tunnel syndrome to...' and 'The purpose of this investigation is to use spectrophotometry to determine variations of skin blood flow response to...'. The use of nominalisation ('likelihood' in the first example; 'variations' and 'response' in the second) involves deagentivisation, rendering the text more compact and more abstract and therefore less LF. Similarly, the frequent use of the passive voice, for example 'this project is being undertaken because we...', 'You are asked to read this patient information sheet carefully before...' runs counter to ethicalness because the passive voice disguises agency.

Compounded noun groups were also frequent across the PIS moves. Compounds are generally more difficult to comprehend than pre- or post-modified nouns; in Danish, they are particularly problematic because they are written in one word as opposed to strings of separate words like in English, and they may be difficult to unpack for lay readers. A few examples will suffice to demonstrate the problem: 'urinaquaporinudskillelsen' (excretion of aquaporins), 'blodgennemstrømningen' (blood flow), 'parathyreoideahormon' (parathyroid hormone), 'hæmpdialysepatient' (patient undergoing haemodialysis) and 'behandlingseffekten' (treatment effect). Hence, extensive nominalisation detracts from the LFPC of the PIS by hampering the processing of meaning.

In conclusion, our analysis of aspects of intra-lingual translation from expert to lay communication identified a lack of ethicalness due, among other things, to the fact that specialised terminology is not translated into lay terminology, the use of officialese in steps requesting consent and the use of nominalisations and passives. These are expert language features and could each have been rendered lexically or lexico-grammatically in more simplified ways. The PISs were insufficiently ethical because meaning was not adequately translated from the expert into the lay mode.

Discourse analysis

In the PISs examined, we consider only Step 1 ('Request participation', introduction) and Step 1 ('State general purpose', purpose). In both moves, but in Step 1 of the purpose move more than in Step 1 of the introduction move, the participant is constructed mainly in ways that are in keeping with the biomedical model, i.e. as a patient who is a member of a group of patients characterised by their disease. This is seen, for example, in 'As you are a dialysis patient, we hereby ask you if you want to participate in ...'

and 'You are kindly requested to participate in a scientific experiment on rectal function in patients with cervical spine dislocation'. In the moves examined, only a single PIS constructs the participant as an individual with a past and a future, thereby broadening the focus in the construction of the reader beyond that of an object of investigation. 'You are soon to have an operation for your blushing and sweats. We are about to investigate the effects of such an operation on those who have it. [...] We therefore want to ask you if you want to participate in this investigation'.

In all of the examples investigated, the reader is constructed as being a layman collaborating with medical professionals.

A key question in the construction of the receiver from an ethical point of view is whether he or she is constructed as an individual with a will of his or her own, in possession of power to decline the invitation to participate. Alarmingly from an ethical point of view, in 5 of the 10 PIS steps, the invitation to participate was formulated more like a command ('You are requested to participate in...' and 'You are being asked to participate in... because...') than as an invitation ('I hereby ask you if you want to...'). Hence, the construction of the reader in these steps clearly negates the ethical paradigm of avoiding coercion.

What this study adds

This chapter demonstrates how aspects of ethicalness surface as a function of the relation between the socio-communicative perspective (context), the formal perspective (conventions and law) and the cognitive perspective (understanding) of the ICD. It suggests that genre theory, SFL, translation theory and discourse analysis individually, and even more so collectively, inform the debate on ethicalness in ICDs by identifying linguistic elements with implications for the LFPC of the PIS. Thus, genre analysis is useful because it adds an important 'text-external' dimension (Bhatia, 2008) to the analysis of HC. This argument is also emphasised by Brown *et al.* (2006: 200): 'It is by attending to the ideas of context and culture [...] that we can build a genuinely "evidence-based" and practice relevant strategy for communication in health care'. Like Clerehan *et al.* (2005, 2006), we could have used SFL to explain how culture and context is manifested in the text. Yet genre theory provides a finer tool for rhetorical structural analysis and allows us to link verbal instantiation to rhetorical function at a fine-meshed, operational level equivalent to the mandated contents elements. The PIS moves were generally found to be 'structurally unethical' by not fronting and clearly voicing the rhetorical purpose of the PIS.

Analysis of field unveiled to what extent the PIS is linguistically (un)ethical at the level of choice of words. The PISs examined preserved identification with the expert environment in which the text is born at the expense of serving the communicative purpose in the lay environment for which its use is intended. There was much register variation within the moves and steps of individual PISs and across the PIS samples, but the register was generally insufficiently lay friendly/patient centred, preventing the PIS from fulfilling its lay-oriented skopos. The PIS samples were also insufficiently ethical from a tenor perspective because they too often failed to disclose the identity of the author in the first move and often used unmitigated requests for participation; using face-threatening acts like requests for IC without face-work flies in the face of the ethical obligation not to coerce.

Translation analysis helped trace particular linguistic elements or remnants of interlingual as well as intra-lingual 'translational deficiencies'like the failure to render specialised concepts in lay terms, the use of officialese in steps requesting consent, the use of nominalisations and the use of the passive voice. Echoing the results of register analysis, translation analysis found that these elements of unethicalness at the lexical and lexico-grammatical levels could have been rendered in the lay mode and hence could have been more ethical by being more comprehensible and assigning agency.

The use of the discourse analytical lens identified some of the constructs and values of the PIS. It showed that the opening moves of the PIS examples analysed fell short of being sufficiently ethical because the reader was almost exclusively discursively constructed as an object belonging to a category characterised in terms of disease, and commanded rather than invited to participate.

What needs to be done

We did not use a new rhetoric approach (Coe *et al.*, 2002) in genre analysis to uncover values and beliefs. Nor does this chapter examine how IC documents are mediated intertextually (following Bhatia, 2008) through relationships with other texts, like the oral part of the process of IC, which could have been both interesting and relevant. Yet, this would have required an ethnographic approach, which was deselected. A fruitful research agenda for health-related genres such as ICDs may encompass continuous exploration of methods for analysing and discussing text-external elements, and the establishment of methodological frameworks spanning methods attending to both text-internal and text-external dimensions.

Clerehan's quantitative measure of 'lexical density' was deselected for the reasons stated above (see 'Informed consent in bioethics research'). We firmly believe that comprehension arises from an interaction between features of the context, the text, the sender and the reader. Moreover, how the investigator explains information about research should not be equated with how the individual processes and interprets that information. Any assessment of readability must therefore be contextual and reader focused (viz. Hirsh *et al.*, 2009) and should involve performance-based user testing of understanding in controlled set-up (Knapp *et al.*, 2011).

Tenor is an important element of linguistic ethicalness, and its importance is likely to vary across moves and steps. Yet, this issue remains to be investigated. Similarly, we did not analyse aspects of personalisation, standing and stance from a tenor perspective, although this could add further insights. Stance would be interesting to study because it shows how much of the content comes across as factual and true (epistemic modality) and how much obligation to do something is put on the reader (deontic modality). We believe that redressing of affronts to face in speech acts like requests for consent through the use of particular combinations of politeness may be just as important in PISs as in other 'functional' genres like business discourse, for example (Pilegaard, 1997b). Yet, this issue needs to be further explored.

We only analysed PISs and not the research protocols on which they were based. We therefore could not analyse all the elements identified by Muñoz-Miquel (2012) or Hill-Madsen (2014), relevant to an intra- or interlingual translation process. Yet analysis of any texts 'preceding' the PIS and the transformation of the contents from the expert context of the research protocol to the lay context of the PIS could reveal aspects of the intra-lingual transformation process to further inform the issue of LFPC.

A text's language shows the author's assumptions about the knowledge (a)symmetry between the writer (expert) and the reader (layman). This implies that preservation of some elements typical of expert communication in the PIS could indicate that the PIS producer believes that the *de facto* intra-lingual translation sufficiently spans the divide between the sender's expert knowledge and the receiver's lay knowledge. However, whether this is indeed so and whether it applies equally to all the investigated elements of expert tenor should be investigated in controlled settings.

Just as a text cannot be analysed in a vacuum to judge its ethicalness, so neither can the discursive construction of the contents and the sender be ignored because the discursive constructions overlap and mutually constitute one another. By only investigating the first moves and their steps, we obtained only a partial view of how the receiver was constructed. Data (not reported here) show that in later PIS moves, the receiver is constructed as a social being having family and friends with whom she/he is invited to discuss participation; and in other statements, for example, addressing the discourse of risk, there are elements pointing towards LFPC as constructing the reader as a person with feelings and hence acknowledging his/her lived experience. A full account of the discursive construction of the receiver therefore requires a full discourse analysis of the entire PIS, which may be undertaken in a future study.

Although much remains to be done, we hope that this chapter sketches avenues for a deeper, interdisciplinary approach informing the discussion of the ethicalness of IC as LFPC.

References

Agre, P., Campbell, F.A., Goldman, B.D., Kass, N. and Boccia, M.L. (2003) Improving informed consent: The medium is not the message. *IRB: Ethics and Human Research Special Supplement* 25 (5), S11–S19.

Anker, A.E., Reinhart, A.M. and Feeley, T.H. (2011) Health information seeking: A view of measures and methods. *Patient Education Counselling* 82, 346–354.

Appelbaum, P.S., Lidz, C.W. and Meisel, A. (1987) *Informed Consent: Legal Theory' and Clinical Practice*. New York: Oxford University Press.

Askehave, I. and Zethsen, K.K. (2003) Communication barriers in public discourse: The patient package insert. *Document Design* 4 (1), 22–41.

Berkenkotter, C. and Huckin, T. (1995) *Genre Knowledge in Disciplinary Communication*. Hillsdale, NJ: Lawrence Erlbaum.

Bhatia, V.K. (2008) Towards critical genre analysis. In V.K. Bhatia, J. Flowerdew and R.H. Jones (eds) *Advances in Discourse Studies* (pp. 166–177). London: Routledge.

Bridson, J., Hammond, C., Leach, A. and Chester, M.R. (2003) Making consent patient centred. *British Medical Journal* 327 (7424), 1159–1161.

Brown, P. and Levinson, S. (1987) *Politeness*. Cambridge: Cambridge University Press.

Brown, B., Crawford, P. and Carter, R. (2006) *Evidence-Based Health Communication*. Maidenhead: Open University Press.

Chewning, B., Bylund, C.L., Shah, B., Arora, N.K., Gueguen, J.A. and Makoul, G. (2012) Patient preferences for shared decisions: A systematic review. *Patient Education Counselling* 86, 9–18.

Christie, F. and Martin, J.R. (1997) *Genre and Institutions: Social Processes in the Workplace and School*. London: Cassell.

Clerehan, R., Buchbinder, R. and Moodie, J.A (2005) Linguistic framework for assessing the quality of written patient information: Its use in assessing methotrexate information for rheumatoid arthritis. *Health Education Research* (20), 334–344.

Clerehan, R. and Buchbinder, R. (2006) Towards a more valid account of functional text quality: The case of the patient information leaflet. *Text Talk* 26, 37–66.

Coe, R.M., Lingard, L. and Teslenko, T. (2002) *The Rhetoric and Ideology of Genre: Strategies for Stability and Change*. Creskill: Hampton Press.

Coulter, A. (2002) *The Autonomous Patient: Ending Paternalism in Medical Care*. London: Nuffield Trust.

Danbury, C., Newdick, C., Lawson, A. and Waldmann, C. (2010) *Law and Ethics in Intensive Care*. Oxford: Oxford University Press.

Den Nationale Videnskabsetiske Komité (2015) Act on Research Ethics. Review of health research projects. Den Nationale Videnskabsetiske Komité. See http://www.cvk.sum.dk/English/actonabiomedicalresearch.aspx (accessed 1 March 2015).

Edwards, S.J.L., Lilford, R.J., Braunholtz, D.A., Jackson, J.C., Hewison, J. and Thornton, J. (1998) Ethical issues in the design of randomized controlled trials. *Health Technology Assessment* 2 (15). See http://www.journalslibrary.nihr.ac.uk/__data/assets/pdf_file/0004/64822/FullReport-hta2150.pdf (accessed 15 February 2015).

Eggins, S. (1994) *An Introduction to Systemic Functional Linguistics*. London: Pinter.

Epstein, R.M. (2000) The science of patient-centred care. *Journal of Family Practice* 49 (9), 805–807.

European Parliament (2001) *Directive 2001/20/EC of the European Parliament and of The Council.* See http://ec.europa.eu/health/files/eudralex/vol-1/dir_2001_20/dir_2001_20_en.pdf (accessed 24 April 2015).

Ezpeleta-Piorno, P. (2012) An example of genre shift in the medicinal product information genre system. *Linguistica Antverpientsia, New Series – Themes in Translation Studies* 11, 173–186.

Faden, R.R. and Beauchamps, T.L. (1986) *A History and Theory of Informed Consent.* New York: Oxford University Press.

Fage-Butler, A. (2013) Improving patient information leaflets: Developing and applying an evaluative model of patient-centredness for texts. *Communication and Medicine* 10 (2), 105–115.

Fairclough, N. (1992) *Discourse and Social Change.* Cambridge: Polity Press.

Flesch, R. (1948) A new readability yardstick. *Journal of Applied Psychology* 32 (2), 221–223.

Fry, E. (1968) A readability formula that saves time. *Journal of Reading* 11 (7), 513–516.

Gunning, R. (1952) *The Technique of Clear Writing.* New York: McGraw-Hill.

Halliday, M.A.K. and Hasan, R. (1989) *Language, Context, and Text: Aspects of Language in a Social-Semiotic Perspective.* Oxford: Oxford University Press.

Hill-Madsen, A (2014) Derivation and transformation: Strategies in lay-oriented intralingual translation. PhD thesis, Aarhus University.

Hirsh, D., Clerehan, R., Staples, M., Osborne, R.H. and Buchbinder, R. (2009) Patient assessment of medication information leaflets and validation of the Evaluative Linguistic Framework (ELF). *Patient Education and Counselling* 77, 248–254.

Hyland, K. (2002) Genre: Language, context and literacy. *Annual Review of Applied Linguistics* 22, 113–135.

Jakobson, R. (1959/2000) On linguistic aspects of translation. In V. Lawrence (ed.) *The Translation Studies Reader* (pp. 113–118). London: Routledge.

Kanj, M. and Mitic, W (2009) *Health Literacy and Health Promotion.* New York: World Health Organisation.

Kickbusch, I. (2001) Health literacy: Addressing the health and education divide. *Health Promotion International* 16, 289–297.

Knapp, P., Raynor, D.K., Silcock, J. and Parkinson, B. (2011) Can user testing of a clinical trial patient information sheet make it fit-for-purpose? A randomized controlled trial. *BMC Medicine* 9, 89.

Lutz, B.J. and Bowers, B.J. (2000) Patient-centred care: Understanding its interpretation and implementation in health care. *Scholarly Inquiry for Nursing Practice* 14 (2), 165–182.

Manson, N. and O'Neill, O. (2011) *Rethinking Informed Consent in Bioethics.* Cambridge: Cambridge University Press.

Marta, J.A. (1996) A linguistic model of informed consent. *Journal of Medical Philosophy* 21 (1), 41–60.

Martin, J.R. (1992) *English Text: System and Structure.* Philadelphia, PA: John Benjamins.

Martin, J.R. (1997) Analysing genre: Functional parameters. In F. Christie and J.R. Martin (eds) *Genre and Institutions: Social Processes in the Workplace and School* (pp. 3–39). London: Cassell.

Muñoz-Miquel, A. (2012) From the original article to the summary for patients: Reformulation procedures in intralingual translation. *Linguistica Antverpientsia New Series – Themes in Translation Studies* 11, 187–206.

National Health Service (2015) Consent and paricipant information. See http://www.hra.nhs.uk/resources/before-you-apply/consent-and-participation/consent-and-participant-information/ (accessed 10 May 2015).

Ness, D.E., Kiesling, S.F. and Lidz, C.W. (2009) Why does informed consent fail? A discourse analytic approach. *Journal of American Academy of Psychiatry Law* 37, 349–362.

Nisbeth Jensen, M. (2013) Translators of patient informatin leaflets: Translation experts or expert ranslators? A mixed methods study of lay-friendliness. PhD thesis, Aarhus Univesity.

Nisbeth Jensen, M. (2015) Optimising comprehensibility in interlingual translation: The need for intralingual translation. In K. Maksymski, S. Gutermuth and S. Hansen-Schirra (eds) *Translation and Comprehensibility* (pp. 163–193). Berlin: Frank & Timme.

Pandiya, A. (2010) Readability and comprehensibility of informed consent forms for clinical trials. *Perspectives in Clinical Research* 1 (3), 89–100.

Pilegaard, M. (1997a) Translation of medical research articles. In A. Trosborg (ed.) *Text – Typology and Translation* (pp. 159–184). Amsterdam: John Benjamins.

Pilegaard, M. (1997b) Politeness in written business discourse. A text-linguistic perspective on request. *Journal of Pragmatics* 28, 223–244.

Pilegaard, M. (2006) Medical writing, revising and editing. In K. Brown (ed.) *Encyclopedia of Language and Linguistics* (pp. 742–745). Amsterdam: Elsevier.

Pilegaard, M. and Ravn, H.B. (2012) Readability of patient information can be improved. *Danish Medical Journal* 59 (5), A4408.

Pilegaard, M. and Ravn, H.B. (2013) Explorative study of patient information sheet: In search of a feasible intervention design to enhance lay friendliness. *Communication and Medicine* 10 (3), 201–211.

Radden, J. and Sadler, J.Z. (2010) *The Virtuous Psychiatrist: Character Ethics in Psychiatric Practice*. New York: Oxford University Press.

Sand, K., Eik-Nes, N.L. and Loge, J.H. (2012) Readability of informed consent documents (1987–2007) for clinical trials: A linguistic analysis. *Journal of Empirical Research on Human Research Ethics* 7 (4), 67–87.

Schenker, Y., Fernandez, A., Sudore, R. and Schillinger, D. (2011) Interventions to improve patient comprehension in informed consent for medical and surgical procedures: A systematic review. *Medical Decision Making* 31 (1), 151–173.

Simons, L., Wren, G. and Buckland, S. (2009) Survey of lay members of research ethics committees (RECs). INVOLVE. National Institute for Health Research. See http://www.invo.org.uk/wp-content/uploads/2012/01/CompleteRECreport2009.pdf (accessed 1 May 2015).

Swales, J.M. (1990) *Genre Analysis: English in Academic and Research Settings*. Cambridge: Cambridge University Press.

Terblanche, M. and Burgess, L. (2010) Examining the readability of patient-informed consent forms. *Journal of Clinical Trials* 2, 157–162.

Terranova, G., Ferro, M., Carpeggiani, C., Recchia, V., Braga, L., Semelka, R.C. and Picano, E. (2012) Low quality and lack of clarity of current informed consent forms in cardiology: How to improve them. *JACC Cardiovascular Imaging* 5 (6), 649–655.

Treweek, S., Lockhart, P. and Pitkethly, M. (2013) Methods to improve recruitment to randomised controlled trials: Cochrane systematic review and meta-analysis. *British Medical Journal Open*. See http://bmjopen.bmj.com/content/3/2/e002360.full (accessed 24 April 2015) doi:10.1136/bmjopen-2012-002360.

Vaughn, L. (2010) *Doing Ethics: Moral Reasoning and Contemporary Issues*. New York: W.W. Norton.

Vermeer, H.J. (1996) *A Skopos Theory of Translation (Some Arguments For and Against)*. Heidelberg: TEXTconTEXT.

WHO (1998) Health promotion glossary. World Health Organisation. See http://www.who.int/healthpromotion/about/HPR%20Glossary%201998.pdf (accessed 19 March 2015).

WHO (2013) Informed consent form templates. See http://www.who.int/rpc/research_ethics/informed_consent/en/ (accessed 11 April 2013).

World Medical Association (2003)WMA Declaration of Helsinki – Ethical Principles for Medical Research Involving Human Subjects. World Medical Association. http://www.wma.net/en/30publications/10policies/b3/ (accessed 12 April 2013).

Zamanian, M. and Heydari, P. (2012) Readability of texts. State of the Art. *Theory and Practice in Language Studies* 2 (1), 43–53.

Zethsen, K.K. (2007) Beyond translation proper. *TTR: Traduction, Terminologie, Rédaction* 20 (1), 281–308.

Zethsen, K.K. (2009) Intralingual translation – An attempt at description. *Meta* 54 (4), 795–812.

6 Exploring the Links Between the Oral and the Written in Patient–Doctor Communication[1]

Vicent Montalt and Isabel García-Izquierdo

In this chapter, we aim to contribute to a holistic and comprehensive view of oral and written modes. From our translation studies perspective, our starting point will be to recognise the possible cultural and conceptual asymmetries between patients and doctors (second section). After noting that more progress has been made in the study and optimisation of oral than of written communication (third section), we will focus on the Calgary-Cambridge Guide (CCG)[2] (fourth section). We analyse the convergences and divergences between consultation, as a genre of oral communication, and contributions based on research into written communication, thus enabling us to put forward proposals that may make it possible to strengthen the links between the two modes of communication, so as to enhance doctor–patient interaction. Our working hypothesis is that some asymmetries may be better resolved through the written mode and that consultations can be optimised by making use of the written mode for particular issues. In this respect, translators and writers may play an important role as mediators between different discourse communities.

Introduction

Communication between health professionals and patients occupies a prominent position in any healthcare system and is conducted both orally and in writing. Many genres, both oral and written, are used in this broad communicative continuum, ranging from guides for patient and informed consent (IC) forms to consultations. Although from a strictly formal point of view, oral genres (consultation, conference lecture, etc.) and written genres (research paper, drug insert) are readily identified, from a communicative perspective the boundary between the oral and written modes is not always easy to determine. For example, an IC (see Pilegaard, this volume) is essentially a written genre that in practice often requires a context of oral interaction in which the health professional adopts the role of an interpreter who facilitates the patient's reading and understanding. Conversely, a medical consultation is fundamentally an oral genre that may make use of the written mode in specific circumstances to facilitate the exchange and understanding of a particular type of information. This multimodal space exhibited by some genres is precisely the area to be addressed in the study presented here.

If we had to identify the core genre (though not, of course, the only genre) that structures and articulates communication between professionals and patients, we could say that it is the medical consultation. It is the most important process of communicative interaction and exchange of information between professionals and patients. It is also the basic tool of healthcare, and, like healthcare itself, it has evolved over time. Pendleton (1984) defines it as 'the central proceeding in medicine', in which the patient goes to the doctor because of some health problem and provides valuable information so that the doctor can arrive at a diagnosis and establish a treatment regimen.

In a consultation, moreover, the patient receives information of vital importance for understanding and adhering to the therapeutic process, avoiding unnecessary anxiety and being able to make informed decisions. This type of information can also come from other oral or written sources beyond the consultation itself, such as oral exchanges with other patients or health professionals, patient blogs, guides for patients, home health manuals (such as the Merck manual), online audiovisual tutorials and popular articles, among others.

The *consultation* genre is currently highly structured and fairly standardised in its practical application. Research carried out over decades has served to provide empirical data on how consultations work and how they are optimised. The Calgary-Cambridge Guide (CCG, to which we will refer later) reflects these advances in improving clinical communication. Since the consultation is a genre that articulates the essential structure of healthcare, we feel that any contribution on the subject of written genres for patients must be consistent with our existing knowledge of oral communication, and particularly consultations. In other words, it is essential to take a holistic view in which the oral mode and the written mode are integrated in a coherent way, obviously taking account of the differences between them and the functions they perform, or can perform, in the wide-ranging and complex continuum of medical and health communication, specifically in clinical contexts. In short, it is a question of exploring and describing the relationship of complementarity between the oral mode and the written mode in the specific case of the consultation: what tasks, communicative actions, types of information, etc., can be better performed in one mode or the other.

In addition to all this, we need to reflect on the context in which the interaction between the patient and the doctor takes place, a context determined both by the difference in the social status of the groups involved, or the fact that they belong to different discourse communities, and by the possible existence of ethnic differences.

This reflection arises from the fact that there is currently an increasing awareness of the importance of language, communication and culture in medical consultations, from the perspective not only of health sciences but also of disciplines such as social psychology, sociology, cultural anthropology, applied linguistics and translation studies.

Cultural Asymmetries Between Health Professionals and Patients

There are two social factors which show the existence of cultural asymmetries in medical and healthcare fields and which, in our view, represent the two sides of the same coin we call culture: first, the democratisation of specialised knowledge and communication between experts and non-experts; and second, the phenomena of migration and mobility in an increasingly interconnected world.

One of the most important issues from a communicative point of view is that health communication takes place between experts and non-experts, united in the same endeavour to improve people's health but separated by whether or not they possess expert knowledge of the subjects in question and by professional codes and roles.

In a society tending towards democratisation of specialised knowledge and the consumption of information of all kinds, communication between experts and non-experts has become an object of research for the disciplines mentioned, some of which have provided conceptual and epistemological frameworks that may be useful to us. Specifically, a notion of interest to us for our project[3] is that of the knowledge community or discourse community. According to Bazerman (2012), from the perspective of text genre theory,

> The term discourse community identifies a grouping of people who share common language norms, characteristics, patterns, or practices as a consequence of their ongoing communications and identification with each other. With respect to writing, the term has been used to point out that different academic collectives write in characteristic registers and genres (see Bazerman 1979; Swales 1990, 1998; Bizzell 1992; Porter 1992; Berkenkotter & Huckin, 1995). The term has been useful in orienting people to a sociological understanding of the varieties of writing done by students, academics and members of other social groupings, often

> differentiated by discipline, kind of institution, and level of education. (Bazerman, 2012: 1)

Patients with a given illness therefore constitute a more or less clearly defined discourse (or knowledge) community, insofar as they share not only norms, characteristics, criteria, concepts, text genres, discursive practices, registers, etc., with respect to communication, but also personal motivations, aims, expectations, concerns about their health, needs for socialisation and empowerment, etc.

Health professionals, for their part, also constitute discourse (or knowledge) communities different from those of patients. Within the category of health professionals, different communities and subcommunities can be distinguished, according to their profession (nurse, physician, surgeon, radiologist, etc.) and medical speciality (cardiology, neurology, paediatrics, etc.). The members of each of these professional communities share conceptual systems, prior knowledge of the discipline, roles in a particular system of organisation and distribution of work, responsibilities, ethical codes, social status, habits of communication, terminological preferences, etc.

This perspective leads us to a view of these discourse communities as distinct socio-professional cultures (the culture of patients with a given illness, the culture of cardiologists, the culture of nurses, etc.), which exist within and outside one particular ethnic and national culture (see Gotti, this volume). In other words, the cultural space of cardiologists goes beyond national boundaries. For example, within the Spanish context, cardiologists and neurologists will share an ethnic and national culture, and a healthcare system, but will have different disciplinary and professional cultures. Conversely, Spanish, Italian and British cardiologists will share far more in terms of discourse and knowledge regarding their discipline and profession than, say, British cardiologists and neurologists.

The second factor we referred to concerns migration and mobility. From the patients' perspective, it is common knowledge that many emigrate to other countries where the language of professional communication is different from their mother tongue and where the system of concepts and values on health and illness may also be different from that of their context of origin.

From the point of view of health professionals, many find work in countries whose language and culture are different from their own. In those contexts, moreover, a foreign professional may have to treat native patients (with whom the usual linguistic and cultural barriers will probably arise) or patients who are themselves foreigners. An example is the Spanish health professionals who move to the United Kingdom to practise and encounter patients of very diverse origins. This is perhaps a less familiar situation, but it is equally important, and above all it exerts an equally powerful influence on the quality of healthcare.

As we can see, defining the notion of culture is a complex task. Katan suggests a definition of culture:

> [...] a system of congruent and interrelated beliefs, values, strategies and cognitive environments which guide the shared basis of behaviour. Each aspect of culture is linked in a [hierarchical] system to form a unifying context of culture, which then identifies a person and his or her culture. (Katan, 1999/2004: 26)

This system of congruent and interrelated beliefs, values, strategies and cognitive environments which guide the shared basis of behaviour can be applied to a particular group of patients with an illness, or of doctors, or of nurses or other health professionals. Thus, in the field with which we are concerned, we think it may be useful to differentiate between ethnic/national culture and socio-professional culture (Montalt-Resurrecció & Shuttleworth, 2012).

If we take culture in ethnic or national terms in healthcare contexts, it constitutes a fundamental notion for the study of communicative interactions between immigrant patients (from countries with different values, beliefs, expectations, concepts, social roles, etc., on health and illness from those they find in the host country) and health professionals in the host culture.

On the other hand, culture understood in socio-professional terms (Montalt-Resurrecció & Shuttleworth, 2012) enables us to study the communicative interactions between patients and health professionals who, despite sharing the values, beliefs, etc., of the same ethnic and national culture, are not members of the same discourse community and therefore belong to different socio-professional cultures.

Here, the notion of socio-professional asymmetries comes into play. They are manifested in differences with regard to prior knowledge of the subject, professional status, social empowerment and ability to participate and make decisions, as well as terminological, phraseological, textual, stylistic, pragmatic, discursive and other preferences and needs.

From our translation studies perspective, García-Izquierdo and Montalt (2013) underline the fact that new social realities have a direct impact on people's lives, especially in sensitive areas such as medicine and healthcare, and make it essential to address the notion of equifunctional and interlinguistic mediation from a broader perspective. In their own words:

> It needs to be borne in mind that as well as situations of intra- and intergeneric symmetry, we may also find ourselves faced with situations of asymmetry produced not only by interlinguistic differences, but

> also by differences in the expectations and needs of receivers of a single language or culture. We therefore need to argue for developing the notion of equigeneric and intergeneric translation, both intra- and interlinguistic, in order to respond to these specific requirements of written communication. (García-Izquierdo & Montalt, 2013: 7–8)

These asymmetries give rise to processes of intralinguistic mediation (and also interlinguistic mediation in the case of foreign patients with little proficiency in the target language and with different conceptual and value systems) based, essentially, on the reformulation and recontextualisation of the knowledge that is the object of exchange and interaction.

One type of asymmetry occurs when the target text is addressed to a group of readers with different needs and expectations and backgrounds. Here, the strategy is heterofunctional or intergeneric translation. Another type of asymmetry occurs when the target language does not yet possess the genre in question. In this case, genres are imported into target languages and cultures through translation (García-Izquierdo & Montalt, 2013: 9).

In short, as we will see in the exploration of the CCG, socio-professional and ethnic-national asymmetries require a detailed analysis of the contexts in which medical communication takes place, as well as a comprehensive approach to the oral and written modes, so as to respond in the best possible way to patients' needs and expectations.

Oral vs Written Communication

In the health context, the relationship between oral and written communication has always been unequally balanced in favour of the former, as witness the rich and longstanding tradition of research on the oral genre we are considering here: the consultation.

In the last five or six decades, many researchers, being aware of its importance for the effectiveness of healthcare, have made contributions designed to improve the consultation process. As early as the 1950s, Michel Balint (1957) conducted the first empirical research on consultations, enabling him to establish the importance both of attentive listening (by the professionals) and of the emotional aspects of the relationship between professionals and patients.

In 1976, Byrne and Long published the book *Doctors Talking to Patients*, which presents research carried out by analysing 2500 consultations recorded in the United Kingdom and New Zealand. This analysis, as well as revealing the influence of personality, both the doctor's and the patient's, on the course of the consultation, enabled them to describe the normal pattern of phases of the consultation, which were established as six in number. Nowadays, Byrne and Long's approach is regarded as a doctor-centred model, quite far removed from current trends, which focus more on the patient.

In 1984, David Pendleton addressed the study of consultations from the perspective of social psychology, using what was then a new technology: video. Pendleton's contributions were to have a major influence on subsequent models of consultation analysis, as is the case with the CCG, to which we will refer later. In 1987, Roger Neighbour, in his book *The Inner Consultation*, described a more patient-centred, five-phase model.

In 1994, in his book *The Doctor's Communication Handbook*, Peter Tate laid more emphasis on the patient's perspective and on his/her world of ideas, concerns and expectations. And in 1989, Stewart and Roter proposed a dual approach to consultation combining the perspective of the patient (illness centred) and that of the doctor (disease centred).

From 2000, the now widely known and used CCG was developed. This is a communication protocol that establishes the progress of the consultation in detail in five main blocks, subdivided, in turn, into over 60 specific steps. We will refer to it in more detail in the next section. In 2002, John Launer put forward a model of a narratological nature whose main objective is to arrive at a proper understanding and construction of the patient's account. In this model, the patient conclusively becomes the main centre of gravity of the interaction involved in the consultation, in keeping with the paradigm of patient centredness.

Although a great deal of work has been done on this oral genre, research on the field of written communication is sparse and in its early stages. This is borne out by the opinions of health professionals (oncologists, nurses, psychologists) and patients expressed in the various focus groups that the Gentt group carried out in the context of the aforementioned research project on written information for cancer patients in which it can be seen, in general terms, that most of the information currently provided to patients is still given orally. It is also confirmed by the great bulk of publications on doctor–patient communication since the 1970s, especially in the English-speaking world. Admittedly, we find some among these that focus on both oral and written communication (e.g. Davis *et al.*, 2002; Weinman, 1990), aiming to put forward rules for reducing the communicative gap whose existence everyone acknowledges, as we saw in the previous section, and even highlighting how effective written communication can be for enhancing understanding and improving patients' adherence to treatments. We also find studies that, despite attempting to address the question of how to improve communication (Roter & Hall, 2006), generally end up turning into theoretical proposals of little practical use, either to patients or to professionals (Conigliaro, 2007: 750). But, above all, we find works that place the emphasis on the (oral) communication skills that professionals need to possess in order to improve communication (e.g. Barca Fernández *et al.*, 2004; Street Jr *et al.*, 2009). Special mention should be made of the studies by Silverman, Kurtz and Draper, published from 1998 onwards

(2004, 2013), which focus on skills for communicating with patients and which led to the *Calgary-Cambridge Guide to the Medical Interview*. This guide, widely used in many clinical and educational contexts, such as the National Health Service in the United Kingdom, was proposed on the basis of empirical work describing specific skills and procedures to guide physicians in their communication processes with patients in consultations. The CCG focuses on expert–lay communication in the oral mode in the clinical setting.

However, some reflections voiced in the Gentt focus groups, both by health professionals and by patients, point to the necessity and the advisability of using written communication to provide certain types of information which, by its nature, will be processed, understood and remembered better if it is transmitted to patients (or their relatives) in the written mode.

We therefore need to determine the amount of information provided to patients, as well as the types of information that will prove most important to them, on the basis of specific, detailed knowledge of reality. The *Calgary-Cambridge Guide to the Medical Interview* sets standards on the competences that health professionals must develop in order for (oral) communication with their patients to be conducted properly. Our analysis consists of mapping the relationship between, on the one hand, the *Calgary-Cambridge Guide to the Medical Interview* and, on the other hand, the contributions that can be made from the field of written communication for patients. The overall aim is to find the points of convergence between the two, where written communication could complement oral and thereby improve the communication process.

An essential concept in this respect, as we will shortly see, will be comprehensibility (readability+legibility) (García Izquierdo & Montalt, forthcoming), as it will help us to explore and strengthen the continuity and complementarity between the oral and the written. So, by thoroughly examining the main stages in the CCG and the specific steps within each stage, we can observe a series of convergences and divergences, and it is useful to understand these and make use of them in order to design and promote high-quality patient-centred communication.

A Case Study: The Calgary-Cambridge Guide

As we saw in the previous section, the CCG was developed by Silverman, Kurtz and Draper. The texts have become established standard texts in communication skills teaching throughout the world, 'the first entirely evidence-based textbooks on medical interviewing'. They explore in detail the specific skills of doctor–patient communication and provide comprehensive evidence of the improvement that those skills can make to health outcomes and everyday clinical practice. They are essential reading for learners at all levels (whether medical students, residents or established practitioners) and for facilitators and programme directors.

The CCG is structured in the following sections:

(1) Initiating the session (introduction; obtains personal data; reasons for the consultation; agenda setting).
(2) Gathering information (encourages the patient to tell his/her story, asks questions and leaves patient time to answer; body language, affect; clarifies statements which are vague; periodically summarises; avoids jargon; encourages the expression of the patient's feelings).
(3) Providing structure (summarises at the end of a specific line of inquiry to confirm understanding; progresses from one section to another using transitional statements).
(4) Building the relationship (demonstrates appropriate non-verbal behaviour; accepts legitimacy of patient's views; uses empathy to communicate; provides support; deals sensitively with embarrassing and disturbing topics; during physical examination, asks permission).
(5) Explanation and planning.
(6) Closing the session (contracts with patient; checks that patient agrees and is comfortable with plan).

These sections are further developed into specific tasks, skills and stages. As we can see, the first four stages concentrate on specific aspects of the consultation, which necessarily involve contact between doctor and patient and therefore oral interaction. However, Section 5, *Explanation and planning*, is particularly relevant to written communication, as we will see. This section is divided into four major blocks (*Providing the correct amount and type of information*; *Aiding accurate recall and understanding*; *Achieving a shared understanding: incorporating the patient's perspective*; and *Planning: shared decision making*), which in turn establish 20 specific actions (numbers 33–52).[4] The CCG contains a further section called *Options in explanation and planning* (numbers 57–71). Point 41 explicitly mentions the advisability of using written communication in the form of texts, diagrams and other visual elements. The need therefore arises for patient and doctor to have access to suitable visual and written resources. It is precisely in this recommendation of the CCG that we find the point of union between the oral mode and the written mode.

Since there is some overlap between the contents of certain items, we will not follow the numerical sequence of the CCG in our analysis but will concentrate instead on those issues that may have a correlate in written communication, in order to assess how the latter could help to improve the communication process. We have organised these issues in three main categories: the patient's perspective; comprehensibility; and information types.

The patient's perspective

Under this heading, we will explore aspects of the CCG that deal with prior knowledge, response, choice, feelings, beliefs and expectations.

In a patient-centred framework of communication, the patient's perspective is fundamental and determines the rest of the communication process. The subsection *Identifying the reason(s) for the consultation* (points 4–7) and the whole sections *Gathering information* (points 8–18) and *Building the relationship* (points 23–32) focus mainly on listening to the patient as an individual, who is the main source of new information for the doctor. Since the patient is a unique individual with a unique experience of illness and health, most of the steps involved in these initial phases of the consultation are inherently oral.

However, a number of principles can be inferred that can be useful when writing and translating for patients in general, such as

- '[...] facilitat[ing] the patient's responses verbally and non-verbally e.g. us[ing] encouragement [...] repetition, paraphrasing, interpretation [...]' (point 11). When addressing patients, writers and translators often seek their readers' involvement and response in the form of participation and adherence. Patients are not passive recipients of information. They are active agents in the communication process.
- 'pick[ing] up verbal and non-verbal cues ([...] speech [...] affect)' (point 12). Non-verbal information such as images of all kinds is crucial in effective communication with patients. Sensitive situations are very frequent, and affective language plays a critical role. Writers and translators need to develop awareness that all words matter, and all words may affect readers in a positive or negative way.
- 'clarify[ing] patient's statements that are unclear or need amplification [...]' (point 13). Although texts address more than one reader, writers and translators of texts for patients should be aware that the experience of the individual patient is unique, and the language with which she or he expresses it is also unique. The underlying principle is that texts should address very specific groups of patients that share part of their experiences.
- '[...] avoid[ing] or adequately explain[ing] jargon' (point 15). Jargon is only shared by the members of the discourse community where it is normally used. Technical terms, when not dealt with adequately, may become communication barriers, create confusion, hinder patients' adherence to treatment and intimidate them.
- 'Accept[ing] legitimacy of patient's views and feelings; [avoiding being] judgmental' (point 26). Although the views and feelings of each individual patient are impossible to know for the writer or translator of written texts, awareness of the existence of cultural and individual differences in feelings and perceptions is paramount.

- 'Us[ing] empathy [...]' (point 28). The power of understanding and imaginatively entering into the feelings and views of the other applies both to the individual and to the culture – ethnic-national groups, specific groups of patients with a particular illness, etc. Writing empathetically facilitates patient's adherence and empowerment, and constitutes one of the big challenges in clinical communication.
- 'Deal[ing] sensitively with embarrassing and disturbing topics and physical pain, including when associated with physical examination' (point 29). Once again, oral communication provides writers and translators with awareness of highly sensitive aspects affecting the patient. Writers and translators should be aware of and responsive to the feelings and emotions of their readers.

The area of the patient's ideas, concerns, expectations, effects – how each problem affects the patient's life (point 17) – is particularly relevant when writing or translating to specific groups of patients. As we have pointed out in the previous paragraphs, cultural asymmetries – both ethnic and socio-professional – play a crucial role in communication and should be dealt with carefully in clinical communication. Point 34 of the CCG focuses on the patient's starting point; specifically, on prior knowledge of the subject and whether or not he or she wishes to receive information. Each patient is a unique individual with particular prior knowledge. However, in the case of specific subgroups of patients (child patients, patients of advanced age, patients with poor literacy, etc.) with the same illness, one might expect that most of them share some knowledge of the subject to a certain degree. That potential shared knowledge would make it possible to formulate written texts for transmitting certain types of more or less standardised information, such as the common side effects of a particular drug. A quite different question is whether or not the patient wishes to receive information, and this is an issue that can only be assessed through interaction with each individual patient.

Drawing on the results of our own research carried out by the Gentt team – in particular the focus groups with patients and health professionals – we can say that the needs for information depend on each individual patient. Furthermore, such needs evolve over time along the illness process. Patients seem to need more information at the beginning of the process, and this need tends to decline as the illness either improves or progresses.

There seem to be different kinds of patients regarding information needs. Some patients are more eager to know and therefore look for information, whereas some other patients prefer not to know beyond what they were told in the consultation. Patients who need additional information tend to resort to the internet or to books. This is especially the case with younger patients. In the case of oncological patients, this behaviour is – according to the psycho-oncologists that took part in the focus groups – counterproductive. It can provoke a great deal of anxiety, which blocks the treatment process due to the high levels of emotional stress.

There are patients who prefer not having additional information beyond that provided by the doctors. Some of these patients only want to know whether or not they are going to die.

According to the specialists, in many cases searching for additional information is a way of gaining a sense of control over their illness process. The more anxiety the patients suffer, the more they feel they are losing control over themselves and their illness. In these cases, the doctors themselves recommend some approved web pages to the patients so that they can satisfy their desire to know more about specific aspects regarding their illness. Generally speaking, however, the specialists think that a patient that needs and looks for a lot of information may become problematic, because the more information the patient has the more difficult it will be for the doctor to control the situation.

Patients' prior knowledge or level of literacy directly affects their ability to understand. There are many studies that highlight how poorly information is suited to the patients' level of literacy (Schillinger *et al.*, 2004) and the need to carry out studies that take patients' opinions into account (e.g. García-Izquierdo & Montalt, forthcoming). In the focus groups carried out by the Gentt team, attention was drawn to the fact that the information included in guides for patients, both that written by nurses and that taken from health websites (nearly always American), does not take account of the patients' level of literacy, and certainly not their expectations. The information, provided by international organisations, was too generic and was sometimes excessively technical, quite remote from the patient's individual experience and lacking in empathy.

Some of the patients that took part in the focus groups expressed their discontent with the way they are treated emotionally. Both patients and psycho-oncologists perceive that doctors sometimes do not show empathy towards patients and do not give them the choice to ask about some issues. Non-verbal communication is fundamental, and sometimes patients do not receive the affection they need. Of course, it all depends on each individual doctor. In addition, there are limits imposed by the amount of time available during the consultation. In the case of patients that would like to ask and know more, the time restrictions during the consultation often make it impossible for the doctor to respond adequately or, indeed, for the patient to even express doubts and ask questions. However, quite often it depends on the doctor's attitude which, in the Spanish context, tends to be paternalistic and assumes that giving information to the patient means anticipating worries and fears. According to some of the experts that took part in the focus groups, it is a social and cultural issue in the sense that Spain is a paternalistic, overprotective country in which self-management of the individual is hardly encouraged. This circumstance would probably explain the fact that there is less written information available to patients than what would be advisable.

The professionals themselves also recognise that although it is better at first not to overwhelm patients with too much information, because of the emotional block they tend to suffer, they may demand to be better informed, depending on their age and level of literacy. One must know how to provide the right information at the right time, and as far as possible the patient should be given joint responsibility, since giving too much data all at once can produce a 'bottleneck' and have an adverse effect on the patient's behaviour. It is up to doctors to decide how and when to administer the information. However, there is no single patient profile: many of them do not want more information than they are given orally, but there may be others (or their relatives) that need to have that additional information in writing, sometimes simply to make sure that they have understood the oral explanation properly. In this sense it is essential to have written information available that can help to expand on the oral information the patient will receive from his or her doctor and not leave it all to the discretion of the specialist.

However, as we have seen, it must be borne in mind that many patients will not understand the information if it is too technical, and professionals are therefore calling for more accessible versions of the guides that facilitate comprehension.

Incorporating the patient's perspective necessarily involves first finding out his/her expectations. It is true that it is difficult to write information for patients that uniformly meet all expectations, but it is also true that if studies of the kind Gentt has carried out are conducted, with questionnaires, interviews and focus groups, the chances of the guides for patients fulfilling the needs of a wider public will be greater. Among the results of the focus groups for patients, we discovered, for example, that their expectations included finding guides or fact sheets on subjects such as care in the home or sexuality and fertility (which are sometimes much more difficult to address in the consultation itself, in front of the specialist) and that they needed those texts to contain more illustrations to help them understand the contents better. Once again, therefore, we should try to ensure that these issues, proposed for oral interaction, should also be considered when producing guides or facts sheets for patients.

Comprehensibility

Under comprehensibility, we cover issues related to structure, language, grammar, visual methods and non-verbal cues. Point 33 refers to giving information in assimilable chunks. This principle clearly applies to written information. It also refers to checking for understanding and using the patient's response as a guide to how to proceed. In oral interaction, checking for understanding is an individual action. In written communication, checking for understanding is paramount. However, comprehensibility tests are rarely carried out with real patients. At most, the texts are formally analysed using readability formulas based on purely quantitative factors, such as the number of words per sentence.

Point 37 partially overlaps with point 33: developing a logical sequence. When developing the logical sequence, it is important to use explicit categorisation or signposting, as indicated in point 38. Once again, this principle is applicable to the written mode. As for using repetition and summarising (point 39), the oral mode requires more repetition than the written mode. Summarising the most important information to facilitate memorisation/retention is essential in writing, where it can be reinforced by graphic elements and other visual techniques. Point 40 touches on one of the issues most strongly emphasised both in oral and in written communication: ease of understanding and avoiding terminology that is too technical and opaque for patients. There are various strategies for avoiding professional jargon and making concepts more comprehensible and transparent for the patient. Some authors refer to de-terminologisation (Campos, 2013; Mayor Serrano, 2008; Montalt-Resurrecció & González Davies, 2007; etc.).

As we can see, this block is the one that can most obviously be linked to written communication, since it refers to questions of readability. In the course of the research project cited in the previous paragraphs, professional linguists and translators were surveyed, and readability tests were carried out on the texts in the corpus of the two hospitals participating in the research (the Hospital Clínico Universitario in Valencia and the Hospital Provincial in Castellón). The working hypothesis formulated in García-Izquierdo and Montalt (forthcoming) is the following: 'drawing on both the quantitative and qualitative analysis we can predict that the corpus of FSP under analysis may be poorly intelligible for the real readership of patients it addresses in the clinical setting we are studying'.

The study shows that the formulation of information for patients needs to be improved – as far as format, legibility and readability are concerned – precisely by improving the organisation and structure of the guides or fact sheets, using repetition and paraphrase techniques, summarising the main issues at the end of each section, using visual methods, etc.

The results of the focus groups reveal that although some progress is being made, most genres of information for patients still use obscure, depersonalised language that lacks empathy. According to the specialists, the information should be precise, specific and easily comprehensible, written in a familiar language. It should be presented in an attractive way by means of images and other visual aids. It should be down-to-earth and should avoid hiding the reality to the patient.

In other words, the proposal for conducting the consultation should exactly correlate with the written information provided to groups of patients. In the case of the written mode, we are speaking of limited, uniform groups of patients, whereas in the oral mode we are thinking of an individual patient.

Types and timing of information

Throughout the CCG, we have identified a number of points regarding types of information that could also be dealt with in the written mode; that is, in combination with the oral mode. Point 35 on the CCG establishes asking patients what other information would be helpful for them, such as aetiology or prognosis. The response to the patient's need for information could be both oral and written. In the case of aetiology and prognosis, individualised information is paramount. However, some of the information bound to be helpful to the patient may be of a more general nature – frequent causes of the disease, statistics about prognosis, etc. – and could be provided in the written mode. One of the additional types of information patients seem to be interested in, at least in our interviews, is nutrition and complementary/alternative medicine such as acupuncture, homoeopathy and naturopathy, as well as emotional and psychological aspects (how to deal with anxiety and stress, how to tell relatives about diagnosis, especially the younger members of the family, etc.).

Points 57 refers to providing clear information about procedures, e.g. what patients might experience, how patients will be informed of results, etc. Although procedures are used according to specific needs of individual patients, they are highly standardised, which means that they can be provided in the written mode. Once the information on procedures has been properly delivered to the patient, they can be related to treatment plans (point 58) orally.

Explaining causation, seriousness and expected outcomes, as well as short- and long-term consequences (point 62), is a crucial aspect of clinical communication between doctor and patient and can be achieved through the oral and the written modes. The oral mode can be used to ensure that the individuality of the problem and situation is always centre stage. The written mode can be used as a complementary resource to add more general information when required.

In general, the experts that took part in the focus groups think that there are a number of general aspects regarding the disease that could be transmitted to the patients through the written mode in a better way. This principle applies to other areas and diseases. For example, when explaining ulcerative colitis to patients, they need to understand what the gastrointestinal tract is and how it works in general terms. Other topics of interest highly relevant to patients are those concerning treatment options and prognosis.

Guides and fact sheets for patients (FSP) have improved over time. Some pharmaceutical laboratories produce and distribute them. However, the distribution of such documents is not widespread, and many patients do not have access to them.

When discussing the pros and cons of different options – e.g. no action, investigation, medication or surgery, non-drug treatment (physiotherapy, walking aides, fluids, counselling, preventive measures) (point 64) – patients may find it useful to have the information in the written mode so that they can retain and analyse it in a better, more attentive way.

Point 65 refers to the steps involved in the treatment, as well as the advantages and side effects. While the treatment plan may be highly individualised, the procedures themselves and the side effects of drugs or other treatments are generally fairly standardised, and it is therefore viable to provide clear, detailed information on them in written form. The advantage of the written mode in this case is that it enables the patient to assimilate the information gradually outside the consultation without having to rely exclusively on his or her attention and memory capacity in relation to what the professional says in the consultation. This capacity may be reduced by the emotional factors typical of such interactions: anxiety, worry, insecurity, uncertainty, etc.

In addition to the sections we have focused on, another area of potential combination of the oral and the written is that regarding safety nets and explanations of possible unexpected outcomes – what to do if the plan is not working, when and how to seek help, etc. – as stated in point 54 (within Section 6, Closing the session). Again, the written mode can provide general information on how to seek help when there are unexpected outcomes.

This section of the CCG (Closing the session) could also be linked to the need for the patient to have sufficient information to be able to make his or her own decisions. A point recognised by the professionals in the focus groups is that information for patients ought to be more strictly regulated by the public authorities and that it should not depend on the goodwill of the professionals involved in the process. There ought to be an interhospital protocol. Once this protocol has been established, however, written information should be put forward as a suggestion, giving the patient more than one possibility to choose from regarding his or her treatment. For example, the psycho-oncologists commented in the focus group that many patients are very interested in alternative treatments, which do not usually form part of the protocol. In addition, alternatives should be suggested in the implementation of the treatment, with patients making their own decisions. In this respect, having written information, as a supplement to oral, could help to set out the various alternatives and enable patients to reflect on their preferences away from the consultation.

Point 36 of the CCG urges doctors to provide information at appropriate times and to avoid giving it prematurely. It will be up to the health professional to decide on this issue in each case. Although this principle of non-anticipation does not affect the preparation of documents, it does have to be taken into account in the distribution of written information. Information overload and distress (point 45) should be avoided by organising the communication process in a holistic way – that is, properly combining the oral and the written modes – and by managing its timing adequately.

Conclusions

Along our analysis of the CCG, we have not been suggesting replacing the oral by the written. Rather, by drawing on the CCG's recommendation of using written information (point 41), we have tried to explore and identify when written information can be introduced and used in combination with the oral mode in the light of our own qualitative investigation on written communication in clinical settings. These investigations are limited to the Spanish context and do not necessarily apply to other contexts. We have used them as a starting point to bridge the gap between the oral and the written in the consultation, a fundamental genre in clinical communication everywhere. Of course, this is only a tentative exploration of the potential interactions between the oral and written that needs further thinking and testing.

One of the main conclusions of our analysis is that our own empirical research is consistent with one of the recommendations of the CCG (point 41) regarding the need to use written and visual information as a complement of the oral consultation. Together with the types of information that can (and probably should) also be conveyed in the written mode, we have also identified a number of principles and criteria regarding the patient's perspective, the timing for the delivery of information and aspects regarding comprehensibility. These principles and criteria can be further investigated and used in educational contexts for the training of medical writers and translators. Translators and writers can play an important role as mediators in healthcare situations in which cultural – both national/ethnic and socio-professional – asymmetries may obstruct efficient communication and health outcomes. Therefore, specialised translator training programmes should take these factors into account and develop educational approaches for emerging communication needs and professional profiles. These approaches should include a solid understanding of the interactions of the oral and the written in healthcare communication as well as interlingual and intralingual strategies in specific genres such as the consultation and the IC.

As we have pointed out, comprehensibility is of critical importance when communicating with patients, but it is not the only issue that matters for improving written communication between doctors and patients in clinical settings. As we have seen, asymmetries of all kinds

– both cultural and individual – and emotional aspects arise in patient–doctor communication. Comprehensibility cannot be reduced to terminological, syntactic and structural aspects of the text. Attitudinal and emotional aspects also play an important role in comprehensibility. The more sensitive and empathetic a text is, the more comprehensible it is bound to be. Conversely, adequate terminological, syntactic and structural choices require awareness, sensitivity, empathy and responsiveness on the part of the writer and translator. In other words, there seems to be a positive feedback process between textual and attitudinal aspects of clinical communication. The opposite is probably true, too. The less awareness on the part of the author of the text, the less adequate the terminological, syntactic and structural choices.

One of the most important things written communication can learn from oral interaction is the importance of empathy and sensitivity. Of course, written communication by its own nature will always be necessarily more detached from the immediate personal experience of oral interaction between an individual patient and an individual doctor. However, we think that there is a lot of room for the improvement of written communication and interaction regarding making texts more sensitive, empathetic and patient centred. The lack of an immediate real context and the communicative distance with the real readers should not prevent writers and translators from understanding and connecting with the real needs and expectations of patients. And a thorough knowledge of the consultation as a clinical genre can be of great help to them in their challenge to optimise clinical communication in the written mode.

In this study, we have shown that there is a rich tradition of research and professional practice in oral communication between doctors and patients from which written communication research can greatly benefit. This long tradition can also learn from a more recent tradition in research in written communication in clinical settings. It would be foolish for both to ignore each other and the area of shared interests. In our view, adopting a holistic view that includes both oral and written communication, as well as other formats and modes (audiovisual, etc.), can contribute to a better understanding of patient–doctor communication. Adopting and adapting some of the elements already established in oral communication – through research and practice – can provide useful concepts and methods for research on written communication. A holistic view of this kind can bring coherence to the rich, broad continuum of healthcare communication.

Further research in this area of enquiry will involve exploring the convergences and divergences, the possibilities and limitations, as well as the complementarity of the oral and written (and audiovisual) modes in order to make the best possible use of the synergies between them in a holistic and patient-centred understanding of clinical communication.

Notes

(1) Research project 'Lenguaje y cultura de la salud' (CSO2014-61928-EXP).
(2) The Calgary-Cambridge Guide was developed from Kurtz *et al.* (1998) and Silverman *et al.* (1998). See http://www.gp-training.net/training/communication_skills/calgary/guide.htm.
(3) FFI2012-34200, Análisis de necesidades y propuesta de recursos de información escrita para pacientes en el ámbito de la oncología (Needs analysis and proposal of written information resources for oncology patients) (Gentt). Ministerio de Economía y Competitividad (Spanish Ministry of Economy and Competitiveness).
(4) See Appendix 1.

References

Balint, M. (1957) *The Doctor, His Patient and the Illness*. London: Pitman Medical. (2nd edn 1964, reprinted 1986). Edinburgh: Churchill Livingstone.

Barca Fernández, I., Miguez, R.P., Martín, P.G., Alarcón, F.F., Lázaro, G.A. and de Castro, F.L. (2004) La información al paciente y su participación en la toma de decisiones clínicas. *Atención Primaria* 33 (7), 361–365.

Bazerman, C. (2012) Issue brief: Discourse communities. See http://www.ncte.org/college/briefs/dc (accessed 20 April 2015).

Byrne, P.S. and Long, B.E. (1976) *Doctors Talking to Patients: A Study of the Verbal Behaviours of Doctors in the Consultation*. London: Her Majesty's Stationery Office.

Campos, O. (2013) Procedimientos de desterminologización: Traducción y redacción de guías para pacientes. *Panace@* 14 (37), 48–52.

Conigliaro, R. (2007) Review of D. Roter & J. Hall (2006) Doctors talking with patients/patients talking with doctors. *Journal of the American Medical Association* 297 (7), 748–752.

Davis, T., Williams, M., Marin, E., Parker, R. and Glass, J. (2002) Health literacy and cancer communication. *Cancer Journal for Clinicians* 52 (3), 143–149.

García-Izquierdo, I. and Montalt, V. (2013) Equigeneric and intergeneric translation in patient-centred care. *Hermes* 51, 39–53.

García-Izquierdo, I. and Montalt, V. (forthcoming) Analysing readability and legibility of fact sheets for patients (FSP) in Spanish in a real clinical setting.

Katan, D. (1999/2004) *Translating Cultures: An Introduction for Translators, Interpreters and Mediators*. London: Routledge.

Kurtz, S.M., Silverman, J.D. and Draper, J. (1998) *Teaching and Learning Communication Skills in Medicine*. Oxford: Radcliffe Medical Press. (2nd edn 2004.)

Launer, J. (2002) *Narrative-Based Primary Care: A Practical Guide*. Abingdon: Radcliffe Medical Press Ltd.

Mayor Serrano, B. (2008) Cómo elaborar folletos de salud destinados a los pacientes. *Cuadernos de la Fundación Dr. Antonio Esteve* 14.

Montalt-Resurrecció, V. and González Davies, M. (2007) *Medical Translation Step by Step. Translation Practices Explained*. Manchester: St. Jerome.

Montalt-Resurrecció, V. and Shuttleworth, M. (2012) Research in translation and knowledge mediation in medical and healthcare settings. *Linguistica Antverpiensia, New Series – Themes in Translation Studies* 11, 9–29.

Neighbour, R. (1987) *The Inner Consultation. How to Develop an Effective and Intuitive Consulting Style*. Lancaster: Kluwer Academic Press.

Pendleton, D. (1984) *The Consultation: An Approach to Learning and Teaching* (No. 6). Oxford: Oxford University Press.

Roter, D. and Hall, J. (2006) *Doctors Talking with Patients/Patients Talking with Doctors: Improving Communication in Medical Visits*. Westport, CT: Praeger.

Schillinger, D.A., Bindman, A., Wang, F., Stewart, A. and Piette, J. (2004) Functional health literacy and the quality of physician–patient communication among diabetes patients. *Patient Education and Counseling* 52 (3), 315–323.

Silverman, J.D., Kurtz, S.M. and Draper, J. (1998) *Skills for Communicating with Patients*. Oxford: Radcliffe Medical Press. (2nd edn 2004, 3rd edn 2013.)

Stewart, J. and Roter, D. (eds) (1989) *Communication with Medical Patients*. Newbury Park: Sage Publications.

Street Jr, R.L., Makoul, G., Arora, N.K. and Epstein, R.M. (2009) How does communication heal? Pathways linking clinician–patient communication to health outcomes. *Patient Education and Counseling* 74 (3), 295–301.

Tate, P. (1994) *The Doctor's Communication Handbook*. Abingdon: Radcliffe Publishing Ltd.

Weinman, J. (1990) Providing written information for patients: Psychological considerations. *Journal of the Royal Society of Medicine* 83, 303–305.

Appendix 1

Calgary Cambridge Guide

Explanation and planning

Providing the correct amount and type of information

33. Chunks and checks: gives information in assimilable chunks; checks for understanding, uses patient's response as a guide to how to proceed.
34. Assesses patient's starting point: asks for patient's prior knowledge early on when giving information; discovers extent of patient's wish for information.
35. Asks patient what other information would be helpful e.g. aetiology, prognosis.
36. Gives explanation at appropriate times: avoids giving advice, information or reassurance prematurely.

Aiding accurate recall and understanding

37. Organises explanation: divides into discrete sections; develops a logical sequence.
38. Uses explicit categorisation or signposting (e.g. 'There are three important things that I would like to discuss. First ...'; 'Now, shall we move on to ...').
39. Uses repetition and summarising to reinforce information.
40. Language: uses concise, easily understood statements; avoids or explains jargon.
41. Uses visual methods of conveying information: diagrams, models, written information and instructions.
42. Checks patient's understanding of information given (or plans made), e.g. by asking patient to restate in own words; clarifies as necessary.

Achieving a shared understanding; incorporating the patient's perspective

43. Relates explanations to patient's illness framework: to previously elicited ideas, concerns and expectations.
44. Provides opportunities and encourages patient to contribute: to ask questions, seek clarification or express doubts; responds appropriately.
45. Picks up verbal and non-verbal cues, e.g. patient's need to contribute information or ask questions; information overload; distress.
46. Elicits patient's beliefs, reactions and feelings re information given, terms used; acknowledges and addresses where necessary.

Planning: shared decision-making

47. Shares own thinking as appropriate: ideas, thought processes, dilemmas.
48. Involves patient by making suggestions rather than directives.
49. Encourages patient to contribute their thoughts: ideas, suggestions and preferences.
50. Negotiates a mutually acceptable plan.
51. Offers choices: encourages patient to make choices and decisions to the level that they wish.
52. Checks with patient: if plans accepted; if concerns have been addressed.

Closing the session

Forward planning

53. Contracts with patient re next steps for patient and physician.
54. Safety nets, explaining possible unexpected outcomes, what to do if plan is not working, when and how to seek help.

Ensuring appropriate point of closure

55. Summarises session briefly and clarifies plan of care.
56. Final check that patient agrees and is comfortable with plan and asks if any corrections, questions or other items to discuss.

Options in explanation and planning

If discussing opinion and significance of problems

57. Provides clear information on procedures, e.g. what patient might experience, how patient will be informed of results.
58. Relates procedures to treatment plan: value, purpose.
59. Encourages questions about and discussion of potential anxieties or negative outcomes.

If discussing opinion and significance of problem

60. Offers opinion of what is going on and names if possible.
61. Reveals rationale for opinion.
62. Explains causation, seriousness, expected outcome, short- and long-term consequences.
63. Elicits patient's beliefs, reactions, concerns re opinion.

If negotiating mutual plan of action

64. Discusses options, e.g. no action, investigation, medication or surgery, non-drug treatments (physiotherapy, walking aides, fluids, counselling, preventive measures).
65. Provides information on action or treatment offered:
    1. Name
    2. Steps involved, how it works
    3. Benefits and advantages
    4. Possible side effects.
66. Obtains patient's view of need for action, perceived benefits, barriers, motivation.
67. Accepts patient's views, advocates alternative viewpoint as necessary.
68. Elicits patient's reactions and concerns about plans and treatments including acceptability.
69. Takes patient's lifestyle, beliefs, cultural background and abilities into consideration.
70. Encourages patient to be involved in implementing plans, to take responsibility and be self-reliant.
71. Asks about patient support systems, discusses other support available.

7 Metaphorical Aspects in Cancer Discourse

Ignasi Navarro i Ferrando

In this chapter, firstly, different perspectives on the notion of metaphor are introduced, along with a characterisation of types within conceptual metaphor theory (CMT), in terms of correspondences between domains. Secondly, cognitive functions of metaphor are discussed, including categorisation and conceptualisation, as well as discourse communicative functions, such as deliberate and novel usage. Then, cognitive and communicative functions of conventional metaphors in a set of genres from medical discourse on cancer are illustrated and discussed. The corpus of data consists of research papers, scientific news notices and press articles. Conclusions are drawn on the characterisation of genres on the basis of metaphorical usage particularly the cognitive and communicative functions of metaphor.

Introduction[1]

The language of medicine, and particularly discourse on diseases like cancer, is generally perceived as a highly literal type of discourse, probably due to the direct link between the human physical body and the contents of the discipline. Notwithstanding this view, the aim of this paper is to unravel certain aspects of the use of metaphors in medical discourse, and more precisely in three particular and distinct genres that frequently instantiate example texts on cancer issues. Thus, the purpose is to undertake comparative analysis between: firstly, medical research papers, written by highly qualified experts and aimed at medical peers as readership; secondly, semi-popularised texts, also addressed to professionals and scientists in general; and finally, press articles, addressed to the general public.

It is assumed as a departing point that metaphor plays an essential role in establishing links between our understanding of the world and scientific language (Brown, 2003). Accordingly, a characterisation of the three genres in terms of metaphor usage and function is pursued, so as to determine the role of metaphorical models in scientific communication.

In recent decades, studies on metaphor and its influence on human understanding have proliferated not only in the fields of linguistics or literary studies, but also in other social sciences. Numerous studies have revealed the power that the use of metaphor may confer on a speaker or writer for purposes of favouring a particular perspective or interpretation. In a pioneering work, Lakoff and Johnson (1980) showed how a great number of metaphorical expressions permeate everyday language and reveal the existence of conceptual models that give coherence to our understanding of recurrent daily situations and everyday life. The expression 'head of state' is a useful illustration. By using it, we map our model of a human being – where 'head' refers to the most important component of our body – onto a model of a country, whose most prominent leader is conceptualised by means of that expression. Lakoff and Johnson revealed that the pervasiveness of metaphorical mappings is not an exclusive feature of literary language, but rather that metaphor occurs as a cognitive mechanism fundamentally necessary for our comprehension of life. According to this view, it may be envisaged that metaphorical models can provide coherence to many spheres of human understanding, from economics, law or politics, to religion or philosophy (see Lakoff & Johnson, 1999), and even science (Brown, 2003; Zeidler, 2013).

The general hypothesis of this approach claims that speakers communicate about these domains by unconsciously using metaphorical language, either in conventional ways or as novel usage. At any rate, that usage is generally non-deliberate, contrary to the traditional claims of the rhetorical view of metaphor, which describes its usage as deliberate and conscious. In this chapter, I suggest that usage may be more or less conscious and deliberate depending on genre and analyse the functions metaphors fulfil in each particular genre.

The Notion of Metaphor

Background

The traditionally accepted idea of metaphor depicts it as a rhetorical device consisting of the substitution of one word or expression for another, so that the process might be understood as a speaker or writer saying one thing and meaning another. That approach is known as the substitution view of metaphor. In a classical work, Whately (1861: 253) defines metaphor as 'a word substituted for another on account of the resemblance or analogy between their significations'. Nevertheless, Black (1955: 280) notices that though the figurative form normally substitutes the literal one, sometimes there is no literal expression at all and a metaphor is just 'the use of a word in some new sense in order to remedy a gap in the vocabulary'. Thus, whereas we may accept that 'king of the jungle' substitutes 'lion' in a figurative sentence like 'the king of the jungle suddenly appeared', a similar substitution mechanism cannot be postulated for expressions like 'the crane lifted two containers'. The name of the bird 'crane' cannot be said to be used instead of anything else, because English has no other name for that type of artefact. Therefore, the first metaphorical use of the word 'crane' – when cranes were invented – did indeed fill the gap in the vocabulary for a new type of machine.

Otherwise, metaphor can be conceived of as the processing of an underlying analogy or similarity between two expressions, an approach known as the comparison view of metaphor. Black also points out the controversy maintained by rhetoricians over the fact that the analogy or similarity is sometimes created by the metaphor rather than expressed by it. Black goes beyond this contention and endorses the interaction view of metaphor, which suggests that two thoughts about different things are active together and supported by a single word or phrase, whose meaning is resultant to their interaction. In this approach, metaphor displays 'fundamentally a borrowing and a sort of intercourse of thoughts, a transaction between contexts, and it therefore requires two ideas which co-operate in an inclusive meaning' (Richards, 1936: 94). Accordingly, the interaction view imposes extension of meaning and certain awareness of that extension on the part of language users (Black, 1955: 286). Metaphor suppresses some details and emphasises others, i.e. organises our view of the target concept ('subsidiary subject') by means of a projection or transfer of the implication system from the vehicle concept ('principal subject'). This vehicle, source or primary concept, provides a set of implications that are projected onto the subsidiary, target or secondary concept, to help language users organise their knowledge of it. The metaphor works by applying to the target concept a set of selected features from the system of associated implications characteristic of the source (vehicle) concept. In addition, the idea of projection between implicational systems and the characterisation of these systems as isomorphic analogue-models is also central to this view (Black, 1962). In a later work, Black (1993) suggests the notions of 'metaphorical statement' and 'metaphor-theme', a distinction that is similar to Lakoff's terms 'metaphorical expression' (e.g. 'we've gone too far') versus 'metaphor' (LOVE IS A JOURNEY).

Lakoff and Johnson (1980) and Lakoff (1993) elaborated a systematisation of Black's proposals that brought about a radical shift in terminology and perspective. According to this view, 'metaphor has come to mean a cross-domain mapping in the conceptual system' (Lakoff, 1993: 203), characterised as a set of ontological correspondences between two domains, where the implicational system of the source domain provides a model for the implications and conceptual relationships in the target domain, albeit under the constraint of the invariance principle that ensures the preservation of the target domain image schematic structure, i.e. its original coherence. Thus, mappings are seen as sets of correspondences that characterise epistemic correlations by mapping knowledge of the source domain onto the way in which we conceive and reason about the target domain. The customary formula to refer to such mappings adopts the form TARGET-DOMAIN IS SOURCE-DOMAIN, as in the LOVE-IS-A-JOURNEY mapping, where the following correspondences provide the mapping configuration:

- The lovers correspond to travellers.
- The love relationship corresponds to the vehicle.
- The lovers' common goals correspond to their common destinations on the journey.
- Difficulties in the relationship correspond to impediments to travel.

(Lakoff, 1993: 207)

In this approach, metaphorical expressions, as encountered in texts and linguistic usage, are linguistic expressions that constitute the surface realisation of mappings between conceptual domains, e.g. *our relationship is on the rocks.* It is crucial to note here that mappings are part of the conceptual system in speech communities and help in the process of understanding and giving coherence to the target domain.

Metaphor patterns

Several patterns of metaphor may be described within the framework of conceptual metaphor theory (CMT; Lakoff & Johnson, 1980). One of these patterns instantiates image metaphors, which map one conventional image onto another and allow for mapping knowledge of the first onto knowledge of the second. Conventional images are structured by image schemas and image metaphors preserve that structure. A typical example of this is TEETH ARE PEARLS.

A second type – ontological metaphors – allows for abstractions such as activities, emotions or ideas to be represented as something concrete, such as an object, substance, container or person. This type of metaphor allows for the conceptual management of components of experience like abstract entities, processes, events, attributes and relations, as concrete objects or tangible substances. Our experience with physical bodies and substances provides a set of patterns such as quantification, categorisation and identification of particular aspects that facilitate conceptual processing. Nominalisation is, therefore, the most basic mechanism for ontological metaphor because it lends to a concept the properties of a thing. A frequent metaphor of this type is MIND IS A CONTAINER. Personification is also a typical scheme of this kind of metaphor, whereby an entity is understood in terms of a human being.

A third pattern is that of orientational metaphors. These metaphors can configure a whole system of concepts on the grounds of another one.

Most of them have to do with spatial orientation (up-down, in-out, near-far, etc.). Things function as they do in our physical environment and orientational metaphors project spatial orientation onto abstract concepts, such as HAPPY IS UP, or SAD IS DOWN. The orientational configuration expressed by the metaphor is not arbitrary, but rather based on our experience of the world through perception and motion. Even so, these metaphors are not necessarily cross-cultural, and variation from culture to culture may exist.

Finally, structural metaphors allow us to build the conceptual configuration of one complex concept or a whole domain in terms of another. Typically, structural metaphors provide a set of correspondences that give way to a set of inference patterns and implications, which facilitate understanding and coherence for the target domain, e.g. ARGUMENT IS WAR.

Functions of metaphor

In addition to conceptual configuration, the communicative aspects in the use of metaphors have also been brought into the spotlight by some authors (Keysar & Glucksberg, 1992; Steen, 2011). A common perspective to approach the different uses and functions of metaphor in discourse consists in paying attention to the intentionality shown by the speaker or writer in the particular use of metaphorical expressions, i.e. their deliberate usage. Steen (2011) suggests that a deliberate use of metaphor implies the speaker's awareness of a cross-domain mapping and an intention to alert the addressee to that mapping, which indicates the presence of a specific rhetorical motivation. The speaker's communicative goal points to changing the addressee's perspective on the current topic in the communicative event by making him/her look at it from the point of view of the source domain in the mapping. This type of usage commonly attains a rhetorical function. The interlocutors process the meaning of a metaphorical speech act as a comparison between the domains. Moreover, in many communicative events, the speaker's intention is to lead the hearer in the process of configuration of both concepts and relationships in the target domain, which reveals a conceptualisation function.

On the other hand, non-deliberate usage results from metaphors that are already conventional in the speech community. Therefore, the meanings activated by the utterance are processed directly as meanings in the target domain; no mappings are processed online in the communicative act. In these cases, the metaphor usually fulfils a categorisation function, since the interlocutors categorise the concepts directly in the target domain.

Metaphor in Science and Medical Discourse

The role of metaphors in science has long been noted as a conceptualisation tool for the elaboration of models in scientific paradigms

(Black, 1962; Gentner & Gentner, 1983; Kuhn, 1962, 1993). It is now widely acknowledged that many theories apply metaphorical models to the explanation of phenomena (Zeidler, 2013) and metaphors have been the object of extensive study in scientific disciplines (Pulaczewska, 1999). Brown (2003: 11–12) points out that 'scientists understand nature largely in terms of metaphorical concepts based on embodied understanding of experience', indeed on very basic and pervasive interaction with the physical world. As a consequence, the understanding of complex systems in nature adapts to conceptual frameworks derived from experiential gestalts. Brown remarks that scientific models and theories are metaphorical constructs used to explain observations, with scientists' access to the world mediated by their perceptual and conceptual reasoning system. In this interface, CMT allows for a view of how scientists reason about and communicate abstract ideas.

As for medicine, discourse has been described from the perspective of genre analysis (Gotti & Salager-Meyer, 2006; Lindblad Yanoff, 1988; Salager-Meyer, 1994; Wilce, 2009; among others; see also Gotti, Montalt & García-Izquierdo and Bellés-Fortuño, this volume) and terminology (Cimino *et al.*, 1994).[2] Gotti and Salager-Meyer (2006) offer a set of studies delving into pragmatics and discourse analysis of oral and written texts. Cimino *et al.* (1994) developed a taxonomy and classification of medical terminology. Dirckx (1983) describes the evolution of medical terminology by providing details on the metaphorical origins of many terms. Esteve (2006) also adopts a diachronic standpoint and offers interesting remarks on etymological metaphors within ophthalmological terminology.

From the cognitive semantics standpoint, Giannoni (2009, 2010) explores the intersection of metaphor and axiological variables in a corpus of English texts comprising abstracts, research articles, book reviews and journal editorials. In particular, this author looks at how high-frequency lexical items employ metaphor to convey the disciplinary values associated with four academic domains: medicine, law, economics and applied linguistics. Their function(s) and distribution are illustrated by relevant examples drawn from the corpus in hand. Giannoni's work focuses on the relation between genre and the diverse functionality of metaphors, which constitutes a valuable contribution to the progressive systematisation of research on the communicative aspects of metaphor.

Apart from Giannoni's contribution, the panorama of systematic accounts of conventional metaphor in medical discourse is still rather unexplored territory. Although some remarks on metaphorical developments in medical language appear in Dirckx (1983), research on metaphorical domains giving coherence to particular semantic aspects of medical discourse is still sparse (see, however, Semino *et al.*, 2004).

In the following sections, evidence is provided of how some conventional metaphors fulfil different cognitive and communicative functions across a set of genres in medical discourse about cancer.

Method and Procedure

In this research, the chosen topic for our focus has a high level of social significance, namely cancer. It occurs frequently across a variety of genres of diverse social scope. A first approach resulting from initial observation of medical texts points to the following hypothesis. Discourse addressed to the general public, like press articles (see Domínguez & Sapiña, this volume), is largely expected to incorporate cognitive models based on culture and everyday experience in order to allow reasoning on cancer and its causes, development and effects. Conversely, specialised formal genres, such as the research article, are expected to reduce the use of metaphor. Finally, genres characterised by an intermediate degree of formality like the science popularisation article, which also shows an intermediate degree of specialisation, are expected to incorporate cognitive models to a lesser degree than press texts.

A sample corpus of texts has been compiled for the purpose of analysis. The texts belong to three different genres that show the degrees of formality and specialisation mentioned above. Two specific keywords were selected so as to guarantee an acceptable homogeneity in content topic despite genre variation. These were 'lymphoma' and 'human immunodeficiency virus (HIV)', with the intention that all the texts in the sample corpus would deal with the topic of lymphomas caused by HIV, which guarantees the expected homogeneity.

Thus, the purpose was to analyse and contrast: firstly, medical research papers in a very formal and conventional style, addressed to peers in the same scientific field; secondly, science news texts also addressed to professionals and scientists but from any discipline; and finally, press articles addressed to a wide audience. Three different genres for analysis were selected due to the hypothesis that different degrees of metaphorisation occur across these genres. As a result, the sample corpus includes eight articles on non-Hodgkin's lymphoma treatment from four specialised medical research journals.[3] These articles were provided by the Department of Haematology-Laboratory at the Catalan Institute of Oncology (ICO), Germans Trias i Pujol Hospital in Badalona, Spain,[4] and cover a time span from 2001 to 2013. In addition, 38 news articles from one of the most popular science news websites, *ScienceDaily* (SD), from a period between June 2006 and October 2014. Finally, 10 press articles from the online edition of the *International New York Times* (INYT) published between April 1994 and March 2015. As for the selection of texts from SD and INYT, an electronic

Boolean search of the keywords was applied, which resulted in the sample described here. In sum, the analysis includes texts from three genres where cancer issues are discussed, and which present three different degrees of formality as well as three different kinds of audience and purpose.

A diagnostic criterion is needed to identify metaphorical expressions, namely where an expression taken literally would pose a logical contradiction or absurdity in the context where it occurs. For that purpose, the metaphor identification procedure (MIP) (Pragglejazz Group, 2007; Steen, 2007; Steen *et al.*, 2010) is applied to the texts under analysis. Steen *et al.* (2010: 15) advise that 'metaphor in discourse can be identified by looking for indirectly used words, which then have to be interpreted by comparison to a more basic sense'. Thus, the method is based on the comparison of contextual meaning with basic meaning for a set of selected items or expressions. The identification of mappings and analogies provides further tools for metaphor analysis.

Once metaphorical language has been identified, the procedure classifies the metaphors into four types, namely ontological, orientational, structural and image metaphors, as described in the second section.

The metaphors described are then analysed in terms of deliberate or non-deliberate usage which in turn depends on the kind of cognitive and discursive functions each metaphor displays. For the metaphorical language identified in this chapter, two cognitive functions are demarcated: conceptualisation versus categorisation. A metaphor fulfils a conceptualisation function when it helps both speaker and hearer in understanding and characterising the cognitive domain constituting the topic of discourse, and the relationships and implications among the concepts of the domain, its frames and scripts. The categorisation function fulfils the purpose of providing categories for entities in the target domain, as is the case when we need to refer to a particular event, process or participant. In addition, other functions relative to rhetoric effects can also be considered.

For the purposes of analysis, attention has been paid only to metaphorical language used to process information about the target domain, HIV-related lymphoma. Other metaphorical expressions pertaining to the conventions of the English language or novel uses employed as stylistic devices have been left out.

Metaphors in Discourse on 'HIV-Related Lymphoma'

Firstly, image metaphors are grounded on the similarity of a single image in the source domain with another image in the target domain, or they just provide the source domain image for conceptualisation of the target concept. This type of metaphor is very expressive because it schematically profiles very concrete aspects of experience. It is used to illustrate particular scenes or qualities of single entities, as in Example 1:

(1) The idea of putting any form of the AIDS virus into people sounds a bit frightening, he acknowledged, but the virus used by his team was '**gutted**' and was no longer harmful. (INYT, 12 September 2011)

The expression 'gutted' recalls the image of an animal that has been emptied of organs so that it can be prepared for food or, in an extended meaning, a room or building that has been emptied for redecoration. In this case, the image of emptied space is transferred to the virus so it is understood to be empty of its previous genetic configuration so that new genetic architecture can be implemented, or just to prevent the effects of those elements that have been removed. The image metaphor helps in understanding what a virus can do or why it should be manipulated. In the context above, the virus has been deprived of its capacity to attack human cells.

Secondly, ontological metaphors are useful to represent an abstraction, activity, emotion or idea as something concrete. In the corpus, the following have been identified.

Quantity is load

The amount of virus or bacteria in a patient or organ is referred to as 'viral load' or 'bacterial load'. The metaphorical expression 'load' helps in the conceptualisation of entities imperceptible to our ordinary senses – such as viruses and bacteria – because it provides a conceptual base, i.e. 'conceptual material which is foregrounded as the locus of attention' (Langacker, 2008: 66). By virtue of the metaphor QUANTITY IS LOAD (Example 2), the presence of viruses or bacteria is understood and categorised as a load or burden because attention is focused on the idea that the patient supports it with effort and suffering, with a strong wish to be free of it, given the negative consequences of retaining it. This metaphor employs a set of other linguistic manifestations that contribute to our understanding of how to deal with viruses. Thus, the metaphorical entailments prompt the use of further expressions, with loads being able to be 'reduced', 'measured', 'carried', 'shed' and so on.

(2) This patient had CD4 lymphocyte count of 6/μL and a HIV **viral load** of 690,000 copies/mL. (*Haematologica*, 2008, 93(1): 149)

Other ontological metaphors found in the corpus point to identifying and categorising particular aspects in the development of the disease.

A damaging occurrence is an event

The basic meaning of 'event' as outlined in dictionaries points at anything that happens, especially something important or unusual, regardless of cognitive domain. In the domain of cancer treatment, 'event' designates any infection or malignancy that occurs at any moment in the period between diagnosis and cure or death. Thus, by means of the metaphor, the term becomes specialised so that only certain types of occurrences are called 'events', namely those that imply any emergence or development of disease, illness, impairment or worsening. In Example 3, cancers are classified as a kind of 'events', in this specialised sense.

(3) ...the incidence and proportion of deaths related to non-AIDS-defining cancers (NADC), mostly infection-related cancers and other non-AIDS-related **events**, is increasing among the HIV-infected population in the cART era,... (*British Journal of Haematology*, 2013, 162: 289)

A survival environment is a niche

Though the original sense of 'niche' is a hollow space in a wall, an extended and conventional meaning of this word is a location suited to a group of organisms of the same type or species, as in an ecological niche. The term in natural science describes the environment where a species has adapted for survival. In the domain of cells and viruses, a type of cell or virus finds the tissue or cell it can live on by means of consuming its proteins or molecules.

(4) the cancer cells find their survival **niche** in the T-cell zones of the lymph nodes and the spleen (*SD*, 3 November 2013)

Cell interaction is crosstalk

The basic sense of the word crosstalk is almost synonymous with 'interference' in the context of spoken communication through technological devices. The main implication points to unwanted information intruding into the communication channel. In the domain of cells, 'crosstalk' is used to indicate that an external biological agent comes into contact with a cell and modifies its molecular configuration or programme by virtue of 'interference' to the normal molecular processes. In addition, in the cellular domain, intervention in the molecular processes may be, and usually is, reciprocal, as seen in Example 5.

(5) Within the **niches**, the lymphoma cells interacted with fibroblastic reticular cells in a reciprocal fashion. This **cross-talk** involved stimulation of the lymphotoxin β receptor (*Blood,* 2011, 118: 831)

Get to infect is homing

The basic sense of the word 'homing' as found in dictionaries relates to animals' special abilities to orient themselves in finding their way home from large distances. What is mapped to the target domain is the attribute 'able to find a home' applied to intrusive or inserted cells. The biological mechanism that allows a cell to home in on another one or on an organ is called receptor, and has to do with enzymatic interaction among cells (see Examples 6 and 7).

(6) Clinical studies have correlated the involvement of chemokine receptors with nodal **homing** of B-cell non-Hodgkin (NHL) and Hodgkin lymphoma.(*Blood*, 2011, 118: 1020)

(7) It is shown that CCR7 indeed regulates **homing** of the lymphoma cells to T cell regions in lymph nodes and the spleen (*Blood,* 2011, 118: 831)

Cell lines are family lines

The source meaning for this metaphorical concept is the succession of persons or things in time. More concretely, the source domain emphasises the sense of generations as a family line because the base of the metaphoric concept consists of cultivating successive generations of cells. Cultivating cell lines aims to keep a line alive as long as possible so that the cells may be used in therapy.

(8) They found that the extract had an inhibitory effect on the growth of lymphoma **cell lines**, while leaving the control healthy cells intact. (*SD* 12 March 2010)

The third class in the metaphor typology is formed by structural metaphors. The most pervasive structural metaphor in cancer discourse is TREATING DISEASE IS WAR. The linguistic manifestation of this metaphor instantiates many expressions depicting the disease, the patient as well as medical care and treatment, as if they were characters in a story. We have named the metaphor following the notational convention in CMT, by using the TARGET DOMAIN IS SOURCE DOMAIN formula, though it is also known as the *war metaphor.*

The war metaphor (see Domínguez & Sapiña, this volume) works in cancer discourse as a complex mapping where many of the concepts that we need to understand the disease, the relationships between them and the frames they configure, find correlative counterparts in the war cognitive domain.

The most relevant correspondence is probably the personification of a tumour, cancer or lymphoma. Literally, cancer is not an entity but a biological process whereby cells produce the wrong substances due to diverse causes – viruses, chemicals or even radiation – and as a consequence, malfunction causes cells to die or mutate. The purpose of the metaphor is therefore to pave the way for more fluid understanding of both the actions to be undertaken and the appropriate attitudes to be adopted towards the disease, by doctors, patients and other participants in the treatment process. Once an entity is conceived of as a person, we are able to reason about it in terms of human relationships. Personification allows for characterisation of an entity through conferring human attributes. In this case, because cancer, as it is understood today, is a relatively new concept in the history of the language, the entity is not only previously unknown in the community culture, but it cannot be perceived with our natural perceptual apparatus either. The target domain entity cannot be seen, heard, smelt or touched in any way by our normal senses. It is evident that the conceptual system needs a structural metaphor so that understanding and communication of the new concept, its development and its impact on our lives can be achieved. Personification allows the conceptual system to incorporate such an entity by conceptualising it as a type of human being. The corpus has revealed a set of collocations, semantic preferences and prosodies that offer a picture of this *personified cancer*. Lymphomas are characterised linguistically as 'malignant', 'aggressive', 'resistant' and 'severe', and so conceptually as *an enemy* whom both patients and doctors have to 'fight'. Doctors aim to make them 'vulnerable'. The personified lymphoma may also be understood as an army committing diverse actions against the patient's body. Lymphomas can 'attack' (develop), 'progress' (extend), 'invade' (proliferate), 'go away from' (remission) and 'return to' (relapse) the patient.

The patient, in turn, is conceived of as a 'fighter' who 'resists' attacks and is viewed as bold and courageous.

Another aspect of the mapping is the portrayal of human cells and the immune system as an army. In the sample data, texts reveal expressions that manifest this conceptualisation such as 'an immune system trained to kill', 'T-cells – a type of white blood cell that fights viruses and tumours', 'genes that program cells to attack cancer', 'cancer-fighting genes' and 'immunoglobulins that fight infections'. Many aspects of this correspondence between body cells and an army are exploited and extended. T-cell activity is linguistically described as the actions of a military corps or army division as in Example 9.

(9) To make T-cells **search out** and destroy cancer, researchers must **equip** them to do several **tasks**: **recognize** the cancer, **attack** it, multiply, and live on inside the patient. (INYT, 12 September 2011)

Source domain concepts like 'search out', 'equip', 'tasks', 'recognise the target' and 'attack', that are attributable to soldiers, contribute to the conceptualisation of the process. Yet it is actually a matter of genetic engineering in its literal form. The source domain provides a previously known set of conceptual frames to enable readers to follow what T-cells do.

The whole process of treatment is expressed and described in terms of a war that includes 'battles' ('T-cells were engaged in a furious battle with his cancer'), strategies ('T-cells search out and destroy cancer') and diverse stages so that victory or defeat is envisaged. Such explicit expressions like 'declare victory' on the part of doctors, or 'the war was on', as reported by a patient, are found in the press corpus.

The following list outlines the conceptual mapping across cognitive domains:

Treating cancer is war

Disease (cancer, lymphoma)	is	the enemy –an army
Infection, development	is	an attack
Worsening	is	progress
Getting better, remission	is	retreat, going away
Relapse	is	return
Patient	Is	fighter
Immune system	is	an army
Immune functions	are	defences
Therapy	is	strategy
Proliferation	is	invasion
Reaction	Is	response
Cells chemical reaction	is	fighting
Immunity	is	resistance (in patient)

The mapping clarifies a set of implications through the personification of disease: a lymphoma is aggressive and severe, and can be highly malignant, invade the body, respond to therapy, attack, go away, return and so forth.

The last in the scheme of metaphor types is orientational metaphor, two of which occur in the sample. The first expresses the control that doctors maintain over patients from diagnosis to cure or death. That control is linguistically referred to as 'follow-up', which suggests that proximity is a hallmark of control. The source domain contributes an attribute of motion (the literal meaning of 'follow') and an orientational clue to proximity and completed contact (up). Altogether, the target domain – doctors controlling treatment – is conceived as doctors following the patient's disease at a very short distance: 'follow-up' implies nearness, as in Example 10.

(10) The median follow-up of living patients in group 1 is 59 months. (*British Journal of Haematology* 112: 909). (March 2001)

The orientational metaphor MORE IS UP (Lakoff & Johnson, 1980) is expressed mainly through the lexical unit 'rise', as in 'rising cancers', 'the rise in non-Hodgkin's lymphoma', 'lymphomas are on the rise' and 'non-Hodgkin's disease has been the third most rapidly rising cancer over the last 20 years'. The quantity of cancer patients in the target domain is correlated with vertical up-down motion in the source domain. Thus, the larger the number of cancer patients the higher the cancer is said to rise, whereas the fewer the number of lymphoma cases the lower it declines. The source domain of the metaphor contributes the expression 'rise', which is predicated on an entity conceived of as in small quantity becoming emergent and increasingly visible.

The orientational metaphor provides a spatial conceptualisation pattern. The metaphor displays an implicational system whereby the entity 'lymphoma' is understood as a living organism that can get up and thereby adopt an influential position in relation to individual human beings as well as the community. The increase is no longer conceived of just as a matter of quantity, as could be expressed literally as in 'the quantity of lymphomas increases'. Rather, the connotation the metaphor adds is a feeling of confrontation against an opponent seen as a threat. The orientational metaphor, therefore, is conceptually compatible with other metaphors like the structural war metaphor and personification (LYMPHOMA/CANCER IS AN ENEMY). In fact, expressions like 'be on the rise' are used in other domains with the meaning 'rebellion', and the increase in the quantity of patients is often expressed metaphorically with 'the rise in cancer', or similar. Conversely, the metaphorical status of the expression 'decline' that refers to the opposite phenomenon, a decrease in the quantity of patients, is not so evident, given that the MIP demands that the contextual meaning and the basic meaning drawn from reference dictionaries should be divergent. Whereas for 'rise' the physical orientational sense of the verb is clearly outlined in dictionaries as its basic sense, distinct from 'increase', for 'decline' the basic dictionary meaning is the 'decrease' sense itself, and no physical sense of movement is central for this word in English.

Genre Variation

Cognitive functions

Two cognitive functions of metaphor, categorisation and conceptualisation are discussed here. For the categorisation function, metaphor is used to create categories in a target domain when no specific vocabulary exists for newly identified phenomena. The creation of terminology for new categories employs this kind of mechanism. The metaphorical terms found in our survey corroborate this claim – niche, viral load, event, crosstalk, homing and cell line. In such, terms based on ontological metaphors 'progressively acquire specialised meanings that are specific to the target domain' (Semino, 2011: 131). This study shows how ontological metaphors fulfil categorisation purposes in the specialised field.

On the other hand, the conceptualisation function is carried out by image and structural metaphors. The process of conceptualisation of the target domain as a complex set of conceptual relationships is led by a structural metaphor where the source domain supplies conceptual material for the understanding of phenomena. Thus, our connecting the concepts of attack, aggressiveness, defence, resistance, fight, victory, defeat and many others offers a model to reason about the treatment of a disease. At the same time, image metaphors offer the possibility of visualising abstract phenomena.

Examining the occurrence of the different types of metaphors in the genres analysed enables an appreciation of clear differences between genres addressed to professionals and genres with general readership. Ontological metaphors are frequent in research papers and scientific magazines, but hardly appear in press articles. Conversely, structural and image metaphors only occur in the press articles in the corpus. Table 7.1 quantifies the linguistic manifestations of ontological, orientational and structural metaphors across the three genres. With the purpose of illustrating the degree of incidence of the structural war metaphor, some of the most idiosyncratic concepts that participate in the mapping have been included in Table 7.1, though other linguistic manifestations of the war metaphor would offer very similar results.

It is observed that the metaphorical expressions that fulfil the categorisation of technical terms hardly appear in press articles. Conversely, the conceptualisation function of structural metaphors is not necessary in specialised research. The conceptualisation function in press articles is enhanced by means of metaphor extensions, namely linguistic expressions

Table 7.1 Linguistic manifestation of ontological, orientational and structural metaphors in three medical discourse genres

Genre (number of words in sample)		*Research paper (28.898)*	*Science News (21.686)*	*Press article (12.734)*
Ontological metaphors	Viral load	10	25	1
	Niche	9	6	0
	Event	25	1	0
	Crosstalk	11	3	0
	Homing	15	8	2
	Cell line	1	3	0
Orientational metaphors	Rise	1	3	8
	Follow-up	29	8	1
Structural metaphor TREATMENT IS WAR	Attack	0	1	12
	Battle	0	0	2
	Fight	0	2	9
	Return	0	0	7
	Invasion	1	2	3

that add new correspondences between target and source domain. Since the structural metaphor is not manifested in research texts, no enhancement through extension takes place in research papers either. This refers to new correspondences like 'cure as victory', 'death as defeat', 'chemical dysfunction as genetic sabotage' and others.

In addition, image metaphors play a descriptive function in non-specialised language. Thus, as an author describes the virus as 'gutted' to signify it is no longer harmful, the source domain image of an emptied body or room helps readers to conceive of an analogous phenomenon through visualisation. Another image metaphor depicts a cure as 'mopping up' cancer cells. Non-specialised genres use the conceptualisation function of structural and image metaphors to guide comprehension of phenomena in a target domain that is too abstract or unknown to the public.

On the other hand, the categorisation function of ontological metaphors helps scientists to refer to relevant and newly described phenomena for which no previous vocabulary exists in specialised discourse.

Communicative functions

Even though cognitive functions of metaphor play a central role in understanding and reasoning, another important aspect in the usage of metaphor in discourse has to do with communicative functions. The standard view in CMT holds that metaphor works conventionally, automatically and unconsciously. However, despite its usage being largely unconscious, language users sometimes decide to employ metaphor deliberately in communication. Moreover, whereas unconscious usage normally occurs as conventional forms and expressions, deliberate metaphor may manifest as novel language, as well as through conventional expressions.

Conscious use of a metaphor requires speaker or writer awareness of the cross-domain mapping, as well as an explicit intention to make that mapping evident to the addressee. Deliberate metaphor usage is described as 'an overt invitation on the part of the sender for the addressee to step outside the dominant target domain of the discourse and look at it from an alien source domain' (Steen, 2011: 37). Conversely, non-deliberate unconscious metaphor does not intend to change the addressee's perspective on a topic in this way, but allows for maintaining the focus of discourse entirely on the target domain.

The observations in this study have revealed that different genres display differences not only in the consciousness of usage (deliberate versus non-deliberate metaphor) but also in the types and degrees of creativity (novel versus conventional language).

Specialised research papers are descriptive texts where language is precise and concise. In the previous section, the predominance of ontological metaphor over other types in specialised research discourse has been illustrated. Ontological metaphors employ conventional linguistic manifestations so their use is mainly unconscious. There is no rhetorical effect in using categories such as 'niche', 'crosstalk' or 'event' in the context of a research paper. These forms have no literal synonyms, but rather they 'fill a gap in the vocabulary'. Since they are conventional in the discourse community, their use as metaphors is non-deliberate and does not involve a call of attention on the addressee about mappings. As a consequence, no mappings are assumed to occur in online cognition, as shown in Examples 11–14.

(11) The **viral load** (measured since 1996 in patients receiving HAART) was determined using NucliSens HIV-1 QT. (*British Journal of Haematology*, 112: 909-915). (March 2001)
(12) In hepatocellular carcinoma, sustained hepatic LT expression in mice causes a sequel of **events**, including acute and chronic liver inflammation, eventually followed by hepatocellular carcinoma. (*Blood*, 2011, 118 (4): 1031)
(13) Within the **niche**, lymphoma cells stimulated a reciprocal cross-talk with gp38_ fibroblastic reticular cells. (*Blood*, 2011, 118 (4): 1020)
(14) The **crosstalk** between lymphoid tumor cells and their microenvironmentprovides pivotal signals for the localization and progression of lymphoidmalignancies. (*Blood*, 2011, 118 (4): 1020)

Orientational metaphors ('follow-up', 'rise') also show a conventional and unconscious usage in specialised texts. In Examples 15 and 16, the writer's intention is by no means to call attention on the imagistic connotations inherited from the physical source domain (see the fifth section), but rather to provide a mere technical description focused on the target domain topic.

(15) A clear relationship has been shown between the **rise** in CD4 lymphocyte counts and the decrease in the incidence of HIV-related lymphomas. (*Haematologica*, 2008, 93 (8): 1129)
(16) At the six-month **follow up**, 89 percent of the patients were either in complete or partial remission after the IT treatment. (*SD*, 16 June 2008)

In contrast to specialised texts, press articles display a diverse array of functions in metaphor usage. The absence of ontological metaphors in the discourse addressed to the general public may be a symptom of their categorisation function only operating within the discourse community of professionals. It fulfils a terminological purpose. As for structural metaphors, their use is generally assumed to be conventional and unconscious, but at the same time they leave the door open for deliberate use and conscious mapping activation. When that is the case, novel unconventional linguistic expressions may occur, which causes a rhetorical effect. Two mechanisms that a writer may use deliberately in order to trigger mapping activation in the addressee have been observed in this chapter. Firstly, the use of inverted commas calls a reader's attention to the source domain of the mapping, as in Examples 17–21.

(17) The idea of putting any form of the AIDS virus into people sounds a bit frightening, he acknowledged, but the virus used by his team was **'gutted'** and was no longer harmful. (INYT, 12 September 2011)
(18) Proteins they release could cause a 'cytokine **storm'.** (INYT, 12 September 2011)
(19) The mutation, known as delta 32, creates CD4 cells – the white blood cells that the virus attacks – lacking a CCR5 surface receptor, the '**door**' that the virus uses to enter the cell. (INYT, 3 July 2013)
(20) ...the hope was that graft-versus-host disease would '**mop up'** all the viral reservoirs. (INYT, 3 July 2013)
(21) If any virus is hiding in the cells' DNA, it is '**spit out**' and can be detected. (INYT, 3 July 2013)

In Examples 17–21, by means of a formal punctuation device, the author shows an overt call for the reader's attention on the mapping. This assertion hints at the explicit author awareness of the mappings and his/her decision to activate the mapping in the addressee's online information processing. The calling for the source domains of 'gutted', 'storm', 'door', 'mop up' and 'spit out' inevitably causes a rhetorical effect because the addressee is led towards a new perspective on the topic. The connotations activated by the cognitive emergence of the source domains produce fresh online mappings that help enhance the conceptualisation of the target domain. Thus, we understand that virus manipulation renders it safe when we conceive of a 'gutted virus', cytokine produces convulsive 'stormy' effects in a human body, viruses have easy access to cells through 'doors', the complete eradication of a virus results in a clean body and certain chemicals make cells expel a virus violently or 'spit it out', as it were.

Another overt indication of online mapping awareness on the part of the writer, indicating deliberate usage, consists in making discourse strategic decisions towards extended use of one metaphor throughout a text. An author intends to cause the progressive emergence of the source domain in the information processes carried out by readers, as they proceed in reading.

An illustration of this strategy is observed in the article 'An Immune System Trained to Kill Cancer' (INYT, 12 September 2011). The source domain 'war' is summoned in the headline by an allusion to 'training to kill', which triggers the personification of both 'immune system' and 'cancer'. Then, the author scatters metaphorical expressions of the war metaphor throughout the text, so that at some point novel expressions start to occur that indeed show novel unconventional correspondences between source and target domain. Thus, at an initial stage the text deploys conventional expressions like 'T-cells fight viruses', 'cells attack cancer' and 'treatment killed off cancer cells'. After several linguistic manifestations, novel enriched expressions appear like 'furious battle', 'search out cancer cells', 'hit the targets', 'genetic sabotage', 'keep leukaemia at bay', 'leukaemia knocked out B-cells' and 'viruses used as carriers'. Finally, creativity flourishes with source internal enhancements like 'innocent targets' to refer to healthy cells that are killed by the immune system itself. The conventional expressions like 'war was on' or 'attack' continue appearing (see Domínguez & Sapiña, this volume), so that the activation of the metaphor in the addressees' minds enables them to process and understand any novel correspondence.

The battery of metaphorical expressions from a single structural metaphor in the same text reveals the author's argumentative strategy. Metaphorical expressions enhance the manifestation of structural metaphor mappings, which guarantees text coherence. The above shows it, presented and understood as a war story. In this line, the creative use of metaphor is apparent in press discourse much more evidently than in the other two genres. Kövecses (2010, 2012) refers to metaphorical creativity as the production of novel or unconventional linguistic manifestations of a conceptual metaphor, based either on the source or target domain. Source domain internal creativity implies that conceptual materials of the source domain that were not conventional previous to the novel usage are employed, in order to represent further insights into the processes perceived in the target domain (for instance, 'genetic sabotage' or 'transplants as a potent weapon [against HIV]').

In the sample of press texts analysed here, the linguistic expression of cancer treatment is enriched with conceptual material from the source domain WAR (source internal creativity). By virtue of this type of creativity a battle can be deemed 'furious', the effect of a therapy based on genetic engineering can be deemed 'sabotage' and undesired effects on the body can be deemed as 'hitting innocent targets'.

On the other hand, 'source external creativity operates within the range of the target domain' (Kövecses, 2010: 665) that welcomes new additional source domains for its conceptualisation. Thus, in the sample text analysed, cells that have been genetically modified are called 'serial killers', so the war metaphor is accompanied by a new metaphor that incorporates a new source domain: the personified entity performing the killing does not discriminate innocent victims from the real enemy, against whom action should be taken. In this case, a new source domain (a murderer who kills serially) adds to the war domain as a supplier of conceptual material for the understanding of a process whereby a type of cells kills another type of cells. The novel linguistic manifestation 'serial killer' activates a source domain in the interlocutors' mind where the killer is a murderer, rather than a soldier. The new phenomenon in the target domain CANCER TREATMENT consists of uncontrolled cells that kill without discrimination, which allows for a new enhancement of the linguistic manifestation of the metaphor, with expressions like 'victim cells'. This 'target induced creativity' (Kövecses, 2010: 665) is pushed by new phenomena in the target domain that draw linguistic manifestations from other culturally familiar domains.

All in all, press discourse allows for deliberate novel metaphorical language together with conventional unconscious metaphor usage. In other contexts, different from the deliberate and immense mapping activation observed above, the war metaphor appears more conventionally and unconsciously, with no online mappings apparently active because of the sparse distribution of metaphorical expressions, as seen in Example 22.

(22) ...a third patient in the study died when his cancer **returned**... (INYT 3 July 2013)

Linguistic and conceptual creativity is one of the differential factors of press texts as compared to science news and research papers, most probably due to the need for rhetorical effects in journalism. In Example 23, another case of target-induced creativity is observed where the effectiveness of a new drug allows for an expressive sports metaphor that highlights this:

(23) Such **home-run drugs** can be approved more quickly and efficiently, he said, with smaller studies than are needed for drugs with less obvious benefits (INYT, 9 December 2012)

As demonstrated, research and press genres differ considerably in terms of the communicative functions of metaphor usage. On the other hand, science news seems to be more narrative based than research papers are, although with the rhetorical effects of journalism very much reduced. What differentiates science news from press is its low degree of creativity in the manifestation of metaphor. Thus, though linguistic manifestations of the three types of metaphor do appear, they are limited to the most conventional forms, as in Examples 24, 25 and 26.

(24) an **aggressive** type of non-Hodgkin's lymphoma, is on the rise, most frequently **striking** men. (SD 9 July 2008)

(25) Non-Hodgkin lymphoma has been on the **rise** over the past few decades as industrial production in the United States has expanded. (SD 29 July 2013)

(26) There the lymphoma cells **crosstalk** with stromal cells (connective tissue cells), which subsequently secrete increased quantities of the chemokines CCL19/CCL21. (SD 17 June 2011)

In light of the data observed, it may be suggested that science news results in a richer genre as far as cognitive functions of metaphor are concerned, but a poorer one in terms of creativity of novel expressions and deliberate usage.

In general terms, discourse addressed to the public incorporates cognitive models based on culture and everyday experience in order to reason about cancer and its causes, development and effects. Accordingly, it shows the highest degree of novel metaphorical expressions and deliberate metaphor usage. Conversely, the most formal genre, the research article, reduces metaphor usage to mere terminological categorisation, which is largely conventional and unconscious within the discourse community. Finally, an intermediate genre like scientific news, which shows an intermediate degree of specialisation, instantiates cognitive models in a way limited to conventional language. This study suggests that metaphor emerges in research papers in the form of specialised terminology, whereas conventional metaphorical mappings provide the basis for a layman understanding of specialised knowledge by means of a larger array of metaphorical expressions.

Conclusions

As Lakoff (1993: 205) propounds, 'as soon as we get away from concrete physical experience and start talking about abstract concepts, emotions or domains that cannot be perceived directly, metaphorical processes are the norm'. Therefore, conventional language includes metaphorical models ineluctably, and some subject matters need metaphor for a proper understanding of their principles and conceptual configurations.

In this context, numerous new terms are metaphorical since their very inception in the language because they employ conceptual material from a known and familiar domain in order to fill gaps in the vocabulary of a new cognitive domain. Aspects of these processes have been illustrated here on a sample of discourse about HIV-related lymphomas. In principle, observations and conclusions may be generalised to discourse on other types of cancer.

As for cognitive functions of metaphor, it seems that similarity relations between source and target domains give rise to technical terms whose metaphorical meaning is grounded on that kind of mapping. Accordingly, specialised research papers incorporate terminology – lexical items – grounded on ontological metaphors. These fulfil a categorisation function by providing terms that fill gaps in specialised vocabulary. On the other hand, structural metaphor, as it manifests in press language, tends to instantiate well-entrenched conventional cognitive models that give coherence to discursive and argumentative aspects. These results explain key aspects of the contrast between the reporting character of research texts and the more argumentative character of press discourse.

With regard to communicative functions, there is variation in the use of particular metaphors across genres that are aimed at different audiences (Semino, 2011), for example, the 'war metaphor'. Users of more specialised genres employ metaphors more unconsciously, while press authors exploit metaphors more deliberately for discursive and argumentative purposes.

The contribution of this research mainly consists in the identification of several frequent metaphors and in signalling some of their functions in medical discourse. This study shows the usual limitations of qualitative analysis. A wider corpus of texts would allow for corroborating the suggestions provided here by means of an extensive quantitative survey. Subsequent research should employ larger corpora for quantitative analysis, so that the initial hypotheses on the discursive functions of metaphor presented here can attain further consolidation.

Notes

(1) Financial support for this research has been granted by Pla 2014 de Promoció de la Investigació de la Universitat Jaume I, Ref. P1·1A2014-02.

(2) There are numerous specialised dictionaries and medical glossaries. See http://www.dmoz.org/Reference/Dictionaries/By_Subject/Medicine/ as an example of a list of online medical dictionaries.

(3) *British Journal of Haematology* © John Wiley & Sons Ltd; *Cancer* © American Cancer Society; *Haematologica. Journal of the European Hematology Association.* Ferrata Storti Foundation; *Blood* © American Society of Hematology.

(4) Special gratitude goes to Dr. José Tomás Navarro from the Catalan Institute of Oncology-Germans Trias i Pujol Hospital, principal investigator of the Lymphoid Neoplasms Group at Josep Carreras Leukaemia Research Institute. See http://www.carrerasresearch.org/ca/Lymphoid_Neoplasms.

References

Black, M. (1954–1955) Metaphor. In *Proceedings of the Aristotelian Society. New Series* (Vol. 55; pp. 273–294). Hoboken, NJ: Blackwell Publishing.

Black, M. (1962) *Models and Metaphors.* Ithaca, NY: Cornell University Press.

Black, M. (1993) More about metaphor. In A. Ortony (ed.) *Metaphor and Thought* (2nd edn; pp. 19–41). New York: Cambridge University Press.

Brown, Th.L. (2003) *Making Truth: Metaphor in Science.* Urbana, IL: University of Illinois Press.

Cimino, J.J., Clayton, P.D., Hripcsak, G. and Johnson, S.B. (1994) Knowledge-based approaches to the maintenance of a large controlled medical terminology. *Journal of the American Medical Informatics Association* 1, 35–50.

Dirckx, J.H. (1983) *The Language of Medicine, its Evolution, Structure, and Dynamics.* Hagerstown, MD: Harper & Row.

Esteve, M.J. (2006) Medical terminology across the centuries: Distinctive features of a chronological study in the field of ophthalmology. *Iberica* 12, 111–126.

Gentner, D. and Gentner, D.G. (1983) Flowing waters or teeming crowds: Mental models of electricity. In D.G. Gentner and A.L. Stevens (eds) *Mental Models* (pp. 99–129). Hillsdale, NJ: Erlbaum.

Giannoni, D.S. (2009) Disciplinary values in English academic metaphors. *Linguistica e Filologia* 28, 173–191.

Giannoni, D.S. (2010) Metaphoric values and disciplinary identity in English research articles. In G. Garzone and J. Archibald (eds) *Discourse, Identities and Roles in Specialized Communication. Linguistic Insights* (Vol. 125; pp. 279–298). Bern: Peter Lang.

Gotti, M. and Salager-Meyer, F. (eds) (2006) *Advances in Medical Discourse Analysis: Oral and Written Contexts.* Bern: Peter Lang.

INYT (International New York Times) See http://www.nytimes.com/.

Keysar, B. and Glucksberg, S. (1992) Metaphor and communication. *Poetics Today* 13 (4), 633–658.

Kövecses, Z. (2010) A new look at metaphorical creativity in cognitive linguistics. *Cognitive Linguistics* 21 (4), 663–697.

Kövecses, Z. (2012) Metaphorical creativity in discourse. In M. Brdar, I. Raffaelli and M. Žic Fuchs (eds) *Cognitive Linguistics between Universality and Variation* (pp. 253–270). Newcastle: Cambridge Scholars Publishing.

Kuhn, Th.S. (1962) *The Structure of Scientific Revolutions.* Chicago, IL: The University of Chicago Press.

Kuhn, Th.S. (1993) Metaphor in science. In A. Ortony (ed.) *Metaphor and Thought* (2nd edn; pp. 533–542). New York: Cambridge University Press.

Lakoff, G. (1993) The contemporary theory of metaphor. In A. Ortony (ed.) *Metaphor and Thought* (2nd edn; pp. 202–251). New York: Cambridge University Press.

Lakoff, G. and Johnson, M. (1980) *Metaphors We Live By.* Chicago, IL: University of Chicago Press.

Lakoff, G. and Johnson, M. (1999) *Philosophy in the Flesh.* New York: Basic Books.

Langacker, R. (2008) *Cognitive Grammar. A Basic Introduction.* Oxford: Oxford University Press.

Lindblad Yanoff, K. (1988) The Rhetoric of Medical Discourse: An Analysis of the Major Genres. See http//:repository.upenn.edu/dissertations/AAI8824810. ProQuest Paper AAI8824810.

Pragglejazz Group (2007) MIP: A method for identifying metaphorically used words in discourse. *Metaphor and Symbol* 22 (1), 1–39.

Pulaczewska, H. (1999) *Aspects of Metaphor in Physics. Examples and Case Studies Resources.* Walter de Gruyter.

Richards, I.A. (1936) *The Philosophy of Rhetoric.* London: Oxford University Press.

Salager-Meyer, F. (1994) Hedges and textual communicative function in medical English written discourse. *English for Specific Purposes* 13 (2), 149–171.

ScienceDaily. See http://www.sciencedaily.com/

Semino, E. (2011) The adaptation of metaphor across genres. *Review of Cognitive Linguistics* 9 (1), 130–152.

Semino, E., Heywood, J. and Short, M. (2004) Methodological problems in the analysis of metaphors in a corpus of conversations about cancer. *Journal of Pragmatics* 36, 1271–1294.

Steen, G. (2007) Finding metaphor in discourse. Pragglejaz and beyond. *Culture, Language and Representation* 5, 9–25.

Steen, G. (2011) The contemporary theory of metaphor – Now new and improved! *Review of Cognitive Linguistics* 9 (1), 26–64.

Steen, G., Dorst, L., Herrmann, B., Kaal, A., Krennmayr, T. and Pasma, T. (2010) *A Method for Linguistic Metaphor Identification. From MIP to MIPVU.* Amsterdam: John Benjamins.

Whately, R. (1861) *Elements of Rhetoric*. Nashville, TN: Southern Methodist Publishing House.

Wilce, J.M. (2009) Medical discourse. *Annual Review of Anthropology* 38, 199–215.

Zeidler, P. (2013) *Models and Metaphors as Research Tools in Science*. Berlin: Lit Verlag.

8 Cancer Metaphors in Sports News: The Match that Must Be Won[1]

Martí Domínguez and Lucía Sapiña

In 1978, Susan Sontag published her book Illness as Metaphor, in which she criticised the use of military metaphors to refer to cancer. This language use, she claimed, contributed to stigmatising both the illness and the ill. Since then, different studies have focused on the use of cancer metaphors. In recent years, the role of the media in the creation and spread of metaphors has also been studied to show how they contribute to the creation of a collective image of cancer. Together with war, sport provides an important metaphor set among those used when writing about cancer. Both metaphors are, in fact, interchangeable in certain contexts due to the elements they connect (e.g. two confronting teams, a playing field, a confrontation). Thus, sports metaphors can work well as an alternative to military metaphors in cancer contexts. The shift might be advisable in cases where patients feel uncomfortable with war metaphors.

This chapter analyses the use of cancer metaphors in the Spanish press through news items regarding three different events related to Futbol Club Barcelona, all of them with a strong impact on society: the announcement in 2011 that player Eric Abidal had a liver tumour; the resignation in July 2013 of Francesc 'Tito' Vilanova as manager, after suffering a relapse of his parotid gland cancer; and Vilanova's subsequent death in April 2014. Our analysis shows that, despite the increase in the use of sports metaphors in cancer news involving prominent sports figures, military metaphors still dominate the journalistic discourse.

Introduction

In the late 1970s, Susan Sontag published her book *Illness as Metaphor* (1978), in which she criticised the use of war metaphors to talk about cancer. This language, she claimed, contributed to stigmatising both the illness and the ill. She predicted, nonetheless, that a better understanding of cancer in the following years, as well as the evolution of treatments, would help to change the language:

> Concepts have started to shift in certain medical circles, where doctors are concentrating on the steep buildup of the body's immunological responses to cancer. As the language of treatment evolves from military metaphors of aggressive warfare to metaphors featuring the body's 'natural defenses' (what is called the 'immunodefensive system' can also – to break entirely with the military metaphor – be called the body's 'immune competence'), cancer will be partly de-mythicized. (Sontag, 1978: 87)

We cannot claim that the concept of 'immune competence' is now in standard use, but some others such as 'immunotherapy' certainly are. However, contrary to Sontag's prediction, the great advancement in cancer knowledge over the last decades has not been reflected in an abandonment of the war metaphor nor, following the author's argumentation, in the demythification of the disease. Her essay, written from the double perspective of writer and patient – Sontag had been diagnosed with breast cancer – has also been questioned by different authors who saw her statements as the fruit of her personal considerations rather than empirical deductions stemming from social research (Clow, 2002; Seale, 2001). Despite those drawbacks, it is commonly acknowledged that her work contributed to drawing attention to the metaphorical language of disease and its effect on patients. In fact, following her work, different studies have delved into the history of cancer metaphors (Jasen, 2009), the advantages and disadvantages of their use (Laranjeira, 2013; Skott, 2002), how they affect the doctor–patient relationship (Casarett *et al.*, 2010; Penson *et al.*, 2004; Reisfield & Wilson, 2004) and the way they are conveyed by the media (Hanne & Hawken, 2007; Seale, 2001; Williams, 2009).

In their classical study *Metaphors We Live By*, Lakoff and Johnson (1980) highlighted the fundamental role of metaphors in the structuring process of the human conceptual system. In conceptual metaphor theory (CMT), metaphors permeate daily life; not only language but also thought and action (Lakoff, 1993). Gibbs (2008) considers the metaphor a fundamental mechanism thanks to which people can conceptualise the world and their own activity. In addition, he claims that metaphors operate both in daily language and in specialised language (see Navarro, this volume). This point is especially interesting because it presents the metaphor as a transverse element between those two language contexts.

Following this framework, in this chapter we try to show how cancer metaphors appear in newspapers when the disease affects famous sports personalities. In order to do that, the metaphors in the Spanish press concerning two cancer cases that have recently affected Futbol Club (FC)

Barcelona – those of the player Eric Abidal and the manager 'Tito' Vilanova – are analysed. Sports news, and especially football information, represents a very specialised context. The world of sports has its own newspapers and programmes and a prominent space in general-interest media. In Spain, and in much of the world, football is considered the king of sports. Footballers and managers are almost stalked by the media. They are media stars, true celebrities with little private life.

Different studies have analysed the role that celebrities with cancer can play in communication efforts regarding the disease (Bell & Seale, 2011; Corbett & Mori, 1999; Hilton & Hunt, 2010) when the media report on their situation. Likewise, researchers have studied their influence in personal risk prevention and perception (Butler Nattinger *et al.*, 1998; Cram *et al.*, 2003; Evans *et al.*, 2014; Kelaher *et al.*, 2008; Lancucki *et al.*, 2012) and the image of death in such media coverage (Ashton & Feasey, 2014). Despite the extensive literature on these questions, very few studies have focused on analysing how celebrities speak about and refer to their disease when they talk to a wide audience.

Metaphors allow abstract, complex or new concepts to be understood in a more familiar and specific way (Domínguez, 2015a; Domínguez *et al.*, 2014; Navarro, this volume; Semino, 2008; Van Dijk, 2003), but they also condition our perspective and spread a specific ideology, as shown by research on critical metaphor analysis (Charteris-Black, 2005; Musolff, 2008). On the other hand, in disease narratives, metaphors can make an experience more comprehensible and connect an individual's illness to collective experience (Skott, 2002). However, as observed by different authors, they can also perpetuate confusion or negative associations in relation to the disease and to other social aspects (Annas, 1995; Campbell, 2011). Hence, our interest in knowing how the abovementioned prominent sportspeople, their doctors and the media that follow them use metaphors to speak about their disease.

The analysis of cancer metaphors in the media in general, and the press in particular, can offer an interesting perspective. Metaphors are clearly not the only narrative tool used by the media, but they can help to analyse how disease is represented (Seale, 2001; Williams, 2009). In her analysis, Williams (2009) classifies all the cancer metaphors found in the newspaper *The Guardian* into 15 groups: cancerous cells are human beings or animals; cancer is a machine, a war, a puzzle, an enigma in a detective story, a tangle, a riddle; carcinogenesis consists of steps or stages; cancer research is a source of light, a movement forward, a quest for the Holy Grail, an archaeological enterprise. She adds one more group, with a single occurrence: cancer is an Achilles' heel. Although Williams identifies the war metaphor as the most common, she claims that a single metaphorical system is not enough to represent the complexity of cancer-related knowledge. In fact, the way in which context provides meaning to metaphors has received much more attention in recent studies (Chiang & Duann, 2007; Domínguez, 2015b, 2015c; Gibbs, 2008; Semino, 2011). Many of these works, based on empirical studies, show the complexity that is associated with general statements on the structure of metaphors in language and thought.

This study analyses the use of cancer metaphors by the Spanish press in the coverage of three cancer events that affected FC Barcelona in the last years: first, the announcement that player Eric Abidal had been diagnosed with a liver tumour (March 2011); secondly, the resignation of Francesc 'Tito' Vilanova as manager of the team (July 2013) after a relapse of the parotid gland cancer he had suffered since November 2011; and, finally, Vilanova's death as a consequence of his disease (April 2014).

We hypothesised that war metaphors still prevail in the public discourse on cancer. Despite the fact that there are more closely related metaphor fields in the context of football – like sports metaphors – the similarities between both fields allow war metaphors to survive in the general perception of cancer.

With the debate about war/sports metaphors in mind, our main goal for the study of the three cases is to analyse the metaphors used to describe the illness, paying special attention to the following research questions (RQs):

RQ1: What are the most common metaphors used when newspapers write about cancer in sports celebrities?
RQ2: What metaphors do these famous patients use most frequently? Which ones do they identify with?
RQ3: What metaphors do doctors use most frequently?
RQ4: Are war metaphors substituted by sports metaphors in the sports context?

Through an analysis of the texts produced by the media and the two sports celebrities themselves, as well as by their direct relatives, we will examine what kind of metaphors are most used to refer to their disease.

Corpus of Analysis: Metaphors We Play By

Background

On 15 March 2011, FC Barcelona player Eric Abidal was diagnosed with a liver tumour after a medical check-up. The following day, the French back-liner went into the team's changing room to explain the diagnosis to his shocked teammates. He successfully underwent surgery the same week in Barcelona's Clinical Hospital. The tumour was removed without any problem and a completely recovered Abidal reappeared on the pitch in early May. However, a year after the diagnosis, the club announced that Abidal had to undergo surgery once again for a liver transplant. His cousin Gerard was to be the donor, according to various newspapers. In April 2012, Abidal had another successful operation, and after a short recovery, he went back to playing an official match with Barcelona (April 2013). Despite his apparent fitness, the club decided not to renew his contract but offered him the position of technical manager of the club's various schools all around the world. After playing for AS Monaco and Olympiacos FC, Abidal finally retired as a player in December 2014.

The case of Vilanova, although coinciding in time, had a very different outcome. On 22 November 2011, months after Abidal's tumour was diagnosed, FC Barcelona announced that Francesc 'Tito' Vilanova, the second manager of the team at the time, had undergone surgery on his parotid gland. Weeks later, he returned to work as usual. In April 2012, manager Pep Guardiola announced his departure from the team to FC Bayern München, and Vilanova took his position as first manager. The doctors assured that he was OK, 'cured and free of the disease'. Nevertheless, in December of that same year, 'Tito' Vilanova relapsed, and a second surgery on his throat was necessary. From January to March 2013, he was treated in New York. In April, he resumed training sessions, and in May, Barcelona managed to win La Liga, but before the summer holidays, Vilanova relapsed once more and had to leave his position as manager. He was 45 years old when he finally died on 25 April 2014.

Methods

We examine three significant events in the developments described above: The first is the club's announcement that the player Eric Abidal had been diagnosed with liver cancer (15 and 16 March 2011). The second is the resignation of FC Barcelona's manager (20 and 21 July 2013). The third and final stage examined is the period between the announcement that Vilanova had passed away and the day of his funeral (25–29 April 2014). We try to include most of the reactions published in the field of sports regarding these events.

We analysed news items from 10 Spanish newspapers: the six most important ones for general information (*El País*, *El Mundo*, *La Vanguardia*, *El Periódico*, *ABC* and *La Razón*) and the four main sports papers (*AS*, *Marca*, *Mundo Deportivo* and *Sport*).

The specialised sports press stands out due to its number of readers. *Marca* is the most read newspaper in the country, even more so than *El País* (the general interest newspaper with the highest number of readers), according to the General Media Study.[2] *As* is the second most read sports newspaper, with *Mundo Deportivo* and *Sport* in the third and fourth positions, respectively. Although all the sports newspapers offer coverage of different teams and sports, *Marca* is considered to be closer to teams from Madrid, especially Real Madrid, while *Sport* is closer to FC Barcelona and other Catalan teams.

Once the dates and the newspapers in the sample were chosen, we carried out a search through *mynews*, a Spanish digital academic database for online and written press. We used the keywords 'Abidal', 'Tito' and 'Vilanova', along with the keyword 'cancer' in news corresponding to the aforementioned dates. Each piece of news or opinion article – along with its headline – was considered a valid registration unit and was classified according to the following criteria: newspaper type, name of the newspaper, information/opinion and whether the text included metaphors about the disease and the sufferers or there was no predominating metaphor type in the text. We have also adapted the Metaphor Identification Procedure (Pragglejaz Group, 2007) to our subject matter. In order to identify the metaphors, the texts in the sample were read carefully. Those lexical units – words or phrases – that could be considered metaphorical were highlighted. After a second reading and interpretation of these units in context, they were classified according to a list of keywords. We established nine categories for the analysis based on previous classifications (Penson *et al.*, 2004; Periyakoil, 2008; Williams, 2009), with some adaptations and extensions to fit the case of study: (1) military, (2) sport, (3) religious, (4) lottery/luck, (5) journey, (6) cleanliness, (7) tragedy, (8) obstacle and (9) other metaphors. In the last category, we included those metaphors that were used scarcely or were very local, like 'Cancer is bullfighting'. When a news item or an opinion article had the same number of metaphors from two different categories (for example, one military metaphor and one sports metaphor), the one appearing in the headline was chosen, as it had been originally highlighted by the newspaper. That way, each news item or analysed unit was assigned to its predominant category.

The categorisation of analysis units into the different groups was verified during the recollection of the sample with an intercoder test carried out by two independent researchers from the field of communication. The reliability index obtained for the intercoder was 0.86 according to the Cronbach's alpha coefficient. For the quantitative analysis, IBM© SPSS Statistics 19 software was used.

Finally, a detailed analysis of different examples from each category was carried out in order to obtain a better understanding of how the news about the illness was transmitted to readers. The Spanish original has been kept for the examples, with our own English translation following each one.

Results: Cancer, the Match that Must be Won

A total of 321 news items were examined, 49 of which corresponded to Abidal's tumour diagnosis, 97 to 'Tito' Vilanova's second relapse and subsequent retirement and 176 to the passing away of the manager. The difference in the amount of instances between the two events can be explained by news values (Wolf, 2000): higher rank or hierarchy of the subject, interruption of the usual course of events, impact on the interest of the nation (the impact when a player is on medical leave is different to when a manager finally gives up his position, especially if it happens in one of the biggest teams in Spanish football), etc. The severity of the event was also more obvious in the case of the manager: his second relapse showed that the usual treatment options had not been successful, while in the case of Abidal, the lack of diagnosis before the doctors performed a biopsy triggered journalistic caution.

Types of metaphors

Metaphors are widely used in the language of sports journalism. More than half of the 321 obtained units, 55% (*N*=178), use different types of metaphors to refer to Abidal's and Vilanova's cancers.

In the results obtained, we can observe an element of geographical proximity. The newspapers that devoted more space to Abidal's and Vilanova's illnesses were the ones from Catalonia, the ones closest to FC Barcelona: *Sport*, *La Vanguardia* and *El Periódico*. Accordingly, they were the ones showing the most extensive use of metaphors to report and explain first, Abidal's illness, then that of Vilanova and, finally, Vilanova's death (see Table 8.1).

Regarding the type of metaphor, the military one was the most widely used in all three events studied, with 43.8% of cases (*N*=78), followed by sports metaphors with 25.2% (*N*= 45) (see Table 8.2). Several headlines reflect the pre-eminence of military and sports metaphors: 'Tito cambia de partido' (Tito starts a different match) (*El País*, 20/7/13), 'Tito reemprende su lucha' (Tito resumes his fight) (*El Mundo*, 20/7/13), 'Apartarse para ganar el partido' (Stepping out to win the game) (*As*, 20/7/13), 'Abidal gana su primera batalla' (Abidal wins his first battle) (*Sport*, 17/3/11), 'Ni un balón atrás…' (Not a single lost ball…) (*Sport*, 20/7/13). We should note that although war metaphors predominate in the first two newspapers

Table 8.1 Number of metaphors by newspaper

Newspaper		*Metaphor*	*Total units*
General-interest press	*El País*	10	20
	El Mundo	16	26
	La Vanguardia	25	44
	El Periódico	19	31
	ABC	13	19
	La Razón	15	21
Sport press	*Marca*	17	21
	As	9	25
	Sport	40	69
	Mundo Deportivo	14	45
Total		178	321

Table 8.2 Types of metaphors

Categories of metaphors	*Frequency*
Military	78 (43.8%)
Sport	45 (25.2%)
Religious	11 (6.1%)
Lottery/luck	4 (2.2%)
Other	16 (8.9%)
Journey	13 (7.3%)
Cleanliness	3 (1.6%)
Tragedy	3 (1.6%)
Obstacle	5 (2.8%)
Total	178 (100%)

analysed regarding Abidal's diagnosis and Vilanova's resignation, the sports metaphor is a close second. Both work in a similar sense, so their similarities (two opposing teams, a playing field or battlefield, the battle/competition that must be won) and their differences (team vs soldiers, cooperation vs obedience) should be considered. In fact, in the sport press, the war metaphor is often used to talk about sports and especially about football: concepts like *defeat, winner, battle, defence, attack* and many others create a wider scenario.

Conversely, in the third event examined, the death of the manager, the difference is much more remarkable; that is, war metaphors are much more common than sports metaphors (see Table 8.3). Furthermore, the metaphor 'Death is the last journey' is closely related to the conventional metaphor 'Life is a journey'. In the journey we call life, death is the last step we take, the final journey, the definitive goodbye. This is reflected in the news items examined, both in the text and in the headlines: 'Francesc "Tito" Vilanova nos dejó ayer para emprender otro camino, el de la vida eterna' (Francesc 'Tito' Vilanova left us yesterday to walk another path, the one of eternal life) (*Sport*, 26/4/14), 'Adiós a Tito Vilanova, un líder natural' (Farewell to Tito Vilanova, a natural leader) (26/4/14), 'El último adiós a Tito' (The last goodbye to Tito) (*Sport*, 29/4/14).

Religious metaphors appear in all three cases. For instance, a chronological review of 'Tito' Vilanova's disease after his resignation as manager of FC Barcelona was titled 'Un calvario de 21 meses' (A 21-month-long *via crucis*) (*El Mundo*, 20/7/13). In 'Cancer is *via crucis*', the source domain refers to the Stations of the Cross, the path of suffering and torture that took Jesus Christ to the cross. By extension, the long treatments that come with cancer, which are usually painful and sometimes even result in death, recall the torture of crucifixion. Nevertheless, religious metaphors would appear more frequently after the former manager passed away, not only referring to the disease but also to the idea of a new *life* in *heaven*, as seen by Christian tradition.

With a lower occurrence, we also find the metaphor of lottery or good/bad luck. An example of this is 'A Tito, al mismo tiempo que se le cumplía el sueño de su vida profesional, le tocaba la otra lotería, esa misma que no da alegría sino tristeza, que está tocando tantos hogares' (While Tito achieved his professional dream, he won the other lottery, the one that brings sadness rather than joy and affects so many homes) (*La Vanguardia*, 21/7/2013). 'Cancer is a lottery' is related to the more conventional and widely used metaphor 'Life is a gamble'. Here, we also find lexical items shared by sports and war metaphors such as *risk*, *gamble*, *win* or *lose*, among others.

Another metaphor refers to cancer as an obstacle in life. If 'Life is a journey', the general experience is that it is one that is full of obstacles. Life is not free from difficulties, and a serious disease like cancer is one of the worst. Moreover, 'Cancer is an obstacle' when it interrupts the life of a young, recognised professional, as in the two analysed cases. Thus, 'Tito' Vilanova's death was commented on in terms of expectations cut short by disease. Spanish tennis player Nicolás Almagro, who heard about Vilanova's passing while playing in the Trofeo Conde Godó tournament against Rafa Nadal, made the following statement at a press conference: 'Es un palo durísimo, una persona que ha hecho un esfuerzo terrible por superar la enfermedad y que cuando parecía que veía la luz al final del túnel, volvía a caer' (It is a hard blow, he made a huge effort to get over the disease and when he could already see the light at the end of the tunnel, he fell again) (*Sport*, 26/4/14). Here, the *obstacle*, cancer, makes the individual fall once and again but, still, he needs to keep going to get out of the tunnel. 'The obstacle is a tunnel' is a variation of 'Cancer is an obstacle'. On entering a tunnel, an individual's perception of the surroundings is limited and he or she is 'trapped'. One can only return to one's initial state of perception after leaving the tunnel. The tunnel is a transitional place; long, dark and claustrophobic in some sense. The light indicates the end, the recovery of the lost perception of the surroundings.

Other metaphors found in the texts analysed referred to cleanliness. The relationship between disease and filth is also quite deeply rooted in different societies. Disease *taints* the body, *spoils* it: 'La enfermedad mancha; no es simpática, ni fotogénica' (Disease smears: it is not pleasant or photogenic) (*El Periódico*, 21/7/14). Sick people lose weight and lose their hair; their skin gets dry. But it is also a *stain* for many societies that keep hiding and ignoring people with serious diseases, even when they are not infectious. Therefore, the pairing cleanliness/filth regarding diseases is deeply rooted in society. We consider that one is cured when one is *clean*. 'Cancer is filth' reflects the idea that cancerous cells have to be *wiped* from the body, the body must be *cleansed*. Hence the following text: 'El cancer ya había aparecido, lo habían limpiado, y había vuelto dos veces' (Cancer had already appeared, they had wiped it out, and it came back twice) (*ABC*, 20/7/13). As with filth, even if you clean, it can *appear* again. Undetected or inactive cancer cells might be present and, eventually, make cancer *reappear*.

Disease can also be understood as a tragedy, one more serious than any other negative experience one could have. We found several expressions of this kind in the sample analysed, both referring to 'Tito' Vilanova's passing away and to Abidal's diagnosis: 'Es un drama' (It is a tragedy) (*ABC*, 26/4/14), 'Drama Abidal. Tiene un tumor en el hígado y será operado el viernes' (Abidal's tragedy. He has a liver tumour and will undergo surgery on Friday) (*Sport*, 16/3/11).

Occasional references to local metaphors (bullfighting) were also found, such as 'Entre el primer y el segundo achaque, Tito Vilanova, que ahora se enfrenta a la tercera cornada del cáncer…' (Between the first and the second relapse, Tito Vilanova, who now faces the third goring of cancer…) (*El Mundo*, 20/7/2013), as well as more literary ones; for instance: 'La enfermedad que lo acosó como un árbol siniestro, y que finalmente ha caído sobre él, interrumpió una carrera y también rompió un equilibrio' (The disease stalked him like a sinister tree, and finally fell onto him, interrupted his career and also broke a balance) (*As*, 26/4/14).

The research questions presented above focused on those metaphors that were used most by the media, patients and their doctors. There are only a couple of instances in which doctors are quoted as part of the coverage of the events analysed; in both of these cases, the war metaphor, which is also the most common one in the media in general, is used (see Table 8.4).

Similarly, people whose comments appeared in newspapers during the different events (players, managers, sport-related personalities, politicians, artists, etc.) used war metaphors in more instances, closely followed by sports metaphors. One explanation for this could be that many of those who were questioned were sports people; both Eric Abidal and 'Tito' Vilanova preferred using sports metaphors. Vilanova wrote and published a public thank-you letter after his resignation, in which he used sports metaphors profusely.

Next, we analyse the metaphors used in the coverage of each event in detail, reflecting the portrayal of cancer in the media.

Eric Abidal's diagnosis

Eric Abidal's diagnosis shocked everyone. Besides, information was scarce at the beginning. People knew he had a tumour but little else was known to the public, so the media was cautious. In fact, headlines, both from the general media and the sport media, were quite prudent. As several

Table 8.3 Type of metaphor by event analysed

	Metaphor type								
	Military	*Sport*	*Religious*	*Lottery/luck*	*Other*	*Journey*	*Cleanliness*	*Tragedy*	*Obstacle*
Vilanova's resignation	30	27	2	4	1	0	3	0	0
Abidal's diagnosis	11	8	1	0	1	0	0	1	1
Vilanova's death	37	10	8	0	14	13	0	2	4
Total	78	45	11	4	16	13	3	3	5

Table 8.4 Types of metaphor used by emitters

		Metaphor type									
		Military	*Sport*	*Religious*	*Lottery*	*Other*	*Travel*	*Cleanliness*	*Tragedy*	*Obstacle*	*Total*
Who speaks	PwC*	0	8	0	0	0	0	0	0	1	9
	Doctors	2	0	0	0	0	0	0	0	0	2
	Media	68	32	11	4	16	13	3	3	4	154
	Others**	8	5	0	0	0	0	0	0	0	13
Total		78	45	11	4	16	13	3	3	5	178

*People with cancer.

**We include statements by people who were interviewed by journalists or whose opinion was expressed on social networking sites and published by the media.

articles pointed out, the diagnosis was not known with certainty: 'Tras la intervención, los especialistas ya podrán sacar conclusiones importantes de su estado y de la gravedad del mismo, aunque los análisis exhaustivos se completarán en un plazo de diez a quince días' (After the intervention, specialists will be able to draw important conclusions concerning his condition and the seriousness of the situation, although exhaustive analyses will be completed in ten to fifteen days) (*Sport*, 17/3/11), 'Una vez extirpado, el tumor será analizado mediante una biopsia para determinar si es de carácter benigno o maligno y, por tanto, aplicar el tratamiento más adecuado. [...] Según fuentes del club azulgrana, existe la fundada esperanza de poder coger a tiempo el tumor, es decir, antes de que se haya extendido' (Once removed, doctors will perform a biopsy on the tumour to determine whether it is benign or malignant and apply the most adequate treatment [...] According to the club there is hope that the tumour will be removed on time, that is, before it has spread) (*Mundo Deportivo*, 16/4/11). In this last text, an ontological metaphor is used to express the anatomical pathology of the tumour: 'The tumour is benign' when it is not dangerous and 'The tumour is malignant' when it is formed by cancerous cells. These terms are often used by both health professionals and by common people. In fact, there is a comparatively worse degree than *malignant*, a degree of extreme seriousness. When the biopsy of the cancerous tumour contains mutations associated with an exaggerated growth and a lower survival prognosis, doctors say 'The tumour is aggressive/very aggressive'. Similarly, this quote expresses another usual metaphor related to the movement or progression of the tumour. If the tumour is localised and can be easily removed, the common phrase used is 'We caught it in time', but if the tumour has spread to other organs, especially to organs that are difficult to operate on, doctors say 'It is too late'.

Furthermore, in the case of Abidal, very few media sources wrote about cancer right away; they had to wait for the result of the procedure, for the sample to be analysed and a clear diagnosis made. Therefore, other words and phrases like 'tumour', 'ailment', 'illness' or 'what ails him' were used. Despite this, the media were aware that it was a serious illness and used both war and sports metaphors to write about it. Among the war metaphors used were 'Solo el tumor ha podido derribar a Abidal' (Only the tumour could knock Abidal down) (*El Periódico*, 16/3/11) and 'La batalla de Abidal' (Abidal's battle) (*Marca*, 16/3/11). The idea that 'Cancer is war' and that the fight starts with the acknowledgement of the disease can be found in texts such as the following one, titled 'Eric ha empezado a curarse' (Eric has started the healing process) (*As*, 16/3/11): 'Siempre en lucha. Pero esa batalla se empieza a ganar el día que eres capaz de decir tengo un tumor. Cuando rompes ese tabú, empiezas a curarte' (Always keep fighting. But you start winning the battle the day you can say I have a tumour. When you break that taboo, you start healing).

Sports metaphors were also very present, although to a lesser degree: 'Eric Abidal, el lateral azulgrana, vive hoy el partido más complicado de su vida' (Eric Abidal, the Barça winger, faces the most difficult game of his life today) (*El Mundo*, 17/3/11); 'Los grandes partidos vienen precedidos de duros entrenamientos, aunque a veces es imposible prepararse para los "choques" que te da la vida. Abidal se enfrentará hoy a su peor rival: el tumor' (Big games are preceded by hard training, although it is sometimes impossible to prepare for the 'clashes' of life. Abidal faces his worst rival today: the tumour) (*La Razón*, 17/3/11).

The remaining metaphors were not very remarkable, at least at that point. However, after his liver transplant and his comeback to professional football, both the media and his own doctors immediately started talking about Abidal's *miracle*.

'Tito' Vilanova's resignation

The case of Vilanova was different because his resignation validated the fears of the press and the fans. Even if one does not have too much information on cancer, it is easy to sense that a second relapse significantly limits the prospects of survival. It was a life-or-death situation, and feelings and metaphors started appearing more frequently.

Although in the whole corpus, war metaphors were more widely used, the cover headlines used more sports metaphors: 'Tito se va para jugar el partido de suvida' (Tito leaves to play the match of his life) (*Marca*, 20/7/14); 'Tito, a la afición: "Sé que este partido no lo juego solo"' (Tito, to the fans: 'I know I'm not playing this match alone') (*El Periódico*, 21/7/14); and 'Tito ante su partido más difícil' (Tito faces his most difficult match) (*La Razón*, 21/7/14). Inside the newspapers, both types of metaphors were used, with a slight preference for war metaphors. The following are some examples: 'Ahora ya sabemos de qué partido hablamos' (We know now what kind of match it is) (*El Periódico*, 20/7/13); 'Vilanova [...] necesita plena dedicación para la batalla' (Vilanova [...] needs full commitment to the battle) (*ABC*, 20/7/13); 'va a tener que enfrentarse a su enfermedad, que ha vuelto de nuevo, sin avisar, casi a traición, aunque ello tiene para Tito una ventaja: la conoce y sabe las armas con que puede combatirla' (he will have to confront his illness, which has come back, without warning, almost sneaking up on him, although that is an advantage for Tito: he knows it and knows the weapons he needs to fight it) (*La Vanguardia*, 20/7/13); 'Vilanova juega la competición más dura, el cáncer, y contra el peor rival, la muerte' (Vilanova plays the hardest competition, cancer, against the worst rival, death) (*El Mundo*, 20/7/13); 'Con Vilanova reclutado de nuevo en su lucha contra el cáncer...' (With Vilanova recruited again in his fight against cancer...) (*El Mundo*, 21/7/13).

In that battle, 'cancer is the enemy'. Cancer is a disease that originates within our body, yet it is *the other*, the *attacker*. An opinion article (*As*,

20/7/13) sends 'los mejores deseos a un hombre joven atacado por una enfermedad traicionera que se resiste a rendirse' (best wishes to a young man attacked by a treacherous disease that refuses to surrender). The disease is interpreted by another journalist as a foreign element, some kind of *alien* that gained access to the body and must be expelled: 'Se trata de que Tito Vilanova se levante y pueda *escupir* el bicho que lleva dentro. Y lo hará. Seguro' (What we need is for Vilanova to stand up and *spit* the bug out of him. And he will. Of course he will) (*As*, 20/7/13).

These kind of comments, although trying to offer comfort to people with cancer, can have the opposite effect, as they show patients how horrible their disease is in other people's eyes. This may be a reason why 'Tito' Vilanova chose the sports metaphor in his farewell letter to the club. Most of the newspapers (the four sports papers and half of the general information newspapers) published it. 'Tito' Vilanova said: 'Sé que este partido no lo juego solo, que formo parte de un club solidario que me ayudará a salir adelante en este largo proceso, como ha hecho hasta ahora' (I know I am not alone in this game, that I'm part of a supportive club that will help me keep going in this long process, as they did before) (*La Vanguardia*, 21/7/13). As can be deduced from these words, certain patients – as well as their families – seem comfortable with sports metaphors. In fact, Vilanova's son retweeted a support message from Risto Mejide, a popular TV host, in his social networks. He said: 'Tito no se retira. Solo se concentra para el partido más importante de su vida #ÀnimsTito' (Tito does not retire. He just concentrates to win the most important game in his life #ÀnimsTito [*Go Tito* in Catalan]) (*El Periódico*, 20/7/13).

The death of a coach

As we mentioned before, war metaphors are still predominant at this point, but disease as a journey and death as the final destination are more present now. Vilanova said goodbye with his resignation – goodbye to his football career; now it was other people who said their final goodbye to the manager. This farewell was definitive. 'Death is a journey', a final farewell, maybe towards oblivion but also maybe towards eternity. The word 'eternal' appeared in several newspapers together with Vilanova's photograph. *Mundo Deportivo*, on the day of the funeral, included a tear falling from the front page headline, which was a simple 'Adiós' (Farewell). The newspaper *La Razón* used the same picture and cover space they had used on 21 July 2013 to announce Vilanova's resignation as manager. The title was now 'Tito Vilanova, adiós a un luchador' (Tito Vilanova, farewell to a fighter) (in the picture, the former manager waved at the supporters during a match). The title mixed the journey and the military metaphors.

After Vilanova's resignation, several front pages used sports metaphors, but after his passing, such metaphors were only used on one front page: 'El último partido de Tito Vilanova' (Vilanova's last match) (*El País*, 26/4/14). Inside the pages of another newspaper, a similar headline was worth noting: 'Tito no pudo remontar el partido' (Tito could not catch up with the score) (*ABC*, 26/4/14). Still on the metaphor 'Cancer is a match,' used previously, the newspaper created a new one, adapting to the new context: 'Death is the last match'. Now the change is not the source domain but the target domain, where cancer has now changed into death. In one case, in fact, a sports metaphor is mixed with a religious metaphor picturing 'Tito' playing on a new pitch in heaven: 'Tito Vilanova saldrá a entrenar por primera vez desde que la muerte le obligara a mudarse de estadio. Lanzará el balón contra las gradas a la espera de que algún ángel despistado se vista de corto y revisará las líneas del campo, embarrado de tanto lagrimón' (Tito Vilanova will go to training for the first time after death forced him to change stadiums. He will throw the ball to the stands, waiting for some absent-minded angel to don the uniform, and will check the pitch lines, muddied with so many tears) (*ABC*, 27/4/14). Metaphors from other sports were also used: 'El sueño interrumpido de un corredor de fondo' (The interrupted dream of a long-distance runner) (*Sport*, 26/4/14); 'Y Tito no pudo correr más. Lo hizo hasta que no le quedaron más fuerzas' (And Tito could run no more. He kept going until he ran out of strength) (*El Mundo*, 26/4/14).

However, as in the other events, war metaphors were predominant: 'Una lucha agónica contra la enfermedad que se lo ha terminado llevando' (An agonising fight against the disease that finally took him) (*El País*, 26/4/14); 'Fue precisamente el curso en el que tuvo que batallar más duro contra su enfermedad' (It was exactly the year he had to fight the most against his disease) (*El Mundo*, 26/4/14); 'Nunca se rindió' (He never surrendered) (*As*, 26/4/14). Battles can also be understood as obstacles. Thus, expressions such as 'Tito luchaba contra gigantes desde hace tiempo' (Tito had fought against giants for a long time) (*As*, 26/4/14) remind us of the unequal strength of the opponents in the biblical tale of David and Goliath. Cancer would be that giant that is almost impossible to defeat alone, as was the case this time.

Cancer is often categorised as an obstacle, bad luck or a mishap, because it interrupts that which was so difficult to achieve. In this case, it refers especially to the fact that, just when Vilanova had achieved his dream of managing the team he had grown up and succeeded in, fortune turned against him: 'Mala suerte: el destino, ese mal nacido que le juega la peor de las pasadas a la mejor de las personas, decidió ensañarse con él' (Bad luck: fate, that swine who plays the dirtiest of tricks on the best of persons, decided to be merciless to him) (*As*, 26/4/14). 'Death is bad luck', but also 'death is an obstacle' that prevents dreams from being fulfilled: 'Una muerte tan sentida y dramática como la de Tito Vilanova, protagonista de un *american dream*' (Such a heartfelt and shocking death as

Tito Vilanova's, main character of a bitter *American dream*) (*La Vanguardia*, 26/4/14).

People with cancer as heroes

The analysis of the metaphors used by newspapers allowed us to confirm other narrative strategies such as attributing extraordinary, heroic features to cancer patients. It is an attempt to position them in the field of legend. This can be seen in Abidal's case but especially in Vilanova's, where premature death contributes to the idea of myth. As the cover of *La Vanguardia* stated the day after the death of the former manager: 'Tito entra en la leyenda' (Tito enters into legend). Some of the information analysed stresses the fact that he started playing when he was young and reached the top through his efforts. But it was then, when he was enjoying his lifelong dream, that cancer struck: 'Creció en el Barça. Se hizo mayor en el Barça y ha hecho grande el Barça. Hoy el Barça es un sueño roto' (He grew up in the Barça. He became an adult in the Barça and he made the Barça important. Today the Barça is a broken dream) (*Sport*, 20/7/13). In this new situation, the readers expect the hero and main character (Vilanova) to be strong enough to fight evil (cancer) and restore the initial situation (recovery and comeback to his dream of managing Barcelona) (Propp, 1985; Seale, 2002a). They highlight his humble origin, his determination to play for FC Barcelona and the obstacles he overcame in order to be the manager of *his* club. When he finally achieved his lifelong *dream*, the disease appears to ruin it. As we have seen, Vilanova was the main character in a 'bitter *American dream*'. He was born in a small village in the north of Catalonia. A young man of humble background, he managed to enter La Masía, FC Barcelona's football school. He befriended Pep Guardiola there, but while the latter went up to the first team, Vilanova went to play for other clubs, mainly in the Spanish second division. In 2002, he became the manager of FC Barcelona's subsidiary. In 2007, Pep Guardiola hired him as a second manager for the main team. The Guardiola–Vilanova duo achieved much in football. After the departure of Guardiola in 2012, Vilanova became the first manager for FC Barcelona. Months later, the club announced the reoccurrence of the parotid gland cancer he had been diagnosed with the previous year.

Vilanova's son declared at his funeral, 'Eras nuestro héroe, nuestro modelo a seguir' (You were our hero, our model to follow) (*El País*, 29/4/14). The president of the club also said 'No eres un hombre normal. Vivir en el recuerdo eterno no está al alcance de cualquiera' (You are not a normal man. Living in eternal memory is not within everyone's reach) (*Sport*, 29/4/14). He even seems to act metaphorically from heaven, like a divinity. Three days after 'Tito' Vilanova's passing, FC Barcelona played against Villarreal CF Barça, lifeless and mournful, was losing 2–0. But Villarreal scored two own goals, and another goal by Messi gave the match to Barcelona. In fact,

Messi even pointed towards the sky after the last goal to dedicate it to Vilanova. The photograph appeared in every newspaper the following day. The headlines toyed with the idea that the former manager had helped from heaven: 'Una Victoria caída del cielo' (A heaven-sent victory) (*El País*, 28/4/14).

The cancer and the FC Barcelona as 'living' entities

As Lakoff and Johnson (1980: 33) suggest, 'perhaps the most obvious ontological metaphors are those where the physical object is further specified as being a person'. In this sense, instead of an object, we find a disease and we see how it is understood as a living being: 'El cáncer vence al exentrenador del Barcelona' (Cancer defeats the former manager of FC Barcelona) (*ABC*, 26/4/14); 'El cáncer se ha llevado a Tito Vilanova pero nunca podrá arrebatárnoslo de nuestros corazones' (Cancer took Tito Vilanova but it cannot snatch him from our hearts) (*Sport*, 26/4/14); 'Cáncer, el apellido de una enfermedad maldita le preparó una estrategia que no pudo contrarrestar' (Cancer, the name of a damned disease, prepared a strategy he could not counter) (*La Razón*, 28/4/14).

Similarly, the team is personified, and Barcelona's team appears as the sufferer. In this sense, the obstacles that the team – as a unit, as a person – had to face over its activity were re-examined. *La Vanguardia* (27/4/14) used the headline 'Un año negro' (A black year), and specified that 'Barcelona está viviendo una temporada repleta de desgracias' (Barcelona is going through a season full of tragedy). The article ended by saying that 'Al Barça le ha mirado un tuerto' (Someone cursed Barça).

But the club also appears as an individual who boldly faces difficulties: 'Ahora [el equipo] tendrá con la dolencia de Abidal el mayor motor para culminar la excelente temporada que lleva a cabo' (With Abidal's ailment, [the team] will now have the best driving force to finish their excellent season) (*El Periódico*, 16/3/11). Several metonymies make it easier to extend the mourning to all the teams and their followers: 'El fútbol pierde a Tito Vilanova' (Football loses Tito Vilanova) (*El Mundo*, 26/4/14); 'Lloramos todos, sin colores' (No colours, we all cry) (*El País*, 26/4/14).

Discussion: War, Mother of All Metaphors

These results prove that the war metaphor still dominates cancer media discourse. Even in a sports context where the sports metaphor is relevant, the military metaphor is not substituted. Both metaphors coexist, although with a small prevalence of the war one. Military metaphors are deeply rooted in the collective imagination to refer to disease. As pointed out by Semino (2008: 100): 'The WAR domain is closely connected with the general SPORTS domain. War and sports are intertwined in cultural history, and are conventionally metaphorised in terms of each other'.

Indeed, in the texts analysed, we can see that they are interchangeable and that war metaphors are used remarkably often in the language of sports.

The newspapers analysed mostly used war metaphors, although sports metaphors were also widely found, especially at the time of 'Tito' Vilanova's resignation as manager of FC Barcelona. Expressions like 'the match of his life' or 'he concentrates to win' recurred. Nevertheless, the results show that war metaphors continue to permeate public cancer discourse. In 'Cancer is war', the enemy *invades, penetrates* the body to *destroy* it and the patient must *fight* to return the blow, *go on the offensive, win battles* and *put an end to the enemy*. War is associated to death and violence and can contribute to increasing the patient's fear and dread of the illness (Periyakoil, 2008).

The 'Cancer is war' metaphor was more common a few years before Sontag's book *Illness as Metaphor* was published. The use of war imagery to describe the disease was not new. It was at the end of the 19th century, however, that the bacilli responsible for tuberculosis and cholera, as well as the organisms responsible for typhus and diphtheria, were discovered. From then on, cancer was the disease that held the most secrets for science (Patterson, 1987). That idea remained until a new euphoria started to appear in American society: Now that the atomic bomb had been developed in record time, now that the moon was 'conquered', we only needed to put the same effort into fighting cancer. In 1971, Nixon talked about the *conquest* of cancer during the signing of the National Cancer Act (Nixon, 1971). The idea that a battle needed to be fought to conquer the disease spread. From that moment on, the war metaphor became part of our cultural legacy (Marshall, 2011).

That, however, does not imply that war metaphors have to be accepted as inevitable for all patients. In an environment where the voice of patients can be heard more and more often, they demand the right to be able to participate in the construction of metaphors referring to their illness. But also among health professionals, the need to start changing the language about cancer is highlighted, suggesting a new usage language befitting the new reality of the disease. As suggested by Slobod and Fuks (2012): 'When medicine is seen as war, patients may believe that becoming healthy is only a matter of "fighting" hard enough. But, who loses when disease "triumphs"?' In addition, in our analysis of newspapers, we found sentences such as the following: 'La consternación popular que ha provocado la derrota en la batalla de Tito contra el cáncer ha superado las expectativas del Barça' (Public dismay following Tito's defeat against cancer exceeded Barça's expectations) (*La Vanguardia*, 29/4/14).

One of the fields in which the concept of a fight is most widely accepted is the world of sports: 'Cancer is a match'. The sports metaphor encourages patients to fight as part of a team, a fact that can comfort them. Responsibility is no longer only on them; it is shared. In this sense, it can be one of the most convincing metaphors for cancer patients

(Campbell, 2011). In fact, the sports metaphor is also used frequently to deal with judicial issues (Archer & Cohen, 1998) or sex and love issues (Palmatier & Ray, 1989).

Evidently, there are similarities between both metaphors ('Cancer is a war' and 'Cancer is a match'). However, while the losers in war are annihilated, captured and humiliated, the loser of a football game may have the feeling of having played better than the opponent, although finally luck favoured the other team. They do not fight to their deaths; it is a competition in which they prove their skill as part of a team. It encourages the patient to keep going, no matter what. The patient, on the other hand, may feel more comfortable with a team strategy, in which decisions are taken through dialogue with the rest of the group. Responsibility is much more diluted. In the sample analysed, we can see examples of this. 'Tito' Vilanova himself stated in his farewell letter to the club: 'Sé que este partido no lo juego solo, que formo parte de un club solidario [...]' (I know I'm not alone in this game, that I'm part of a supportive club [...]). Sports, and especially football, are seen as team activities. This fact can be more stimulating for the patient, as the prevailing message is not that they have to win the game alone, but precisely that not everything depends on them and they have the best players to face the challenge. Although some authors think the sports metaphor also polarises the result in terms of winners and losers (Periyakoil, 2008), defeat in war usually implies humiliation, loss of freedom and even death; a sports defeat, however, is substantially less dramatic.

Reisfield and Wilson (2004) maintain that no metaphoric concept is inherently good or bad; that all of them are contextual and have strengths and weaknesses. In the same way, Semino (2008: 178) thinks that 'By and large, metaphors are not intrinsically harmful or beneficial, especially at the level of the individual: what matters is how a metaphor is used, and the extent to which individuals are free and able to select the metaphors that work best for them'. Nonetheless, in the war metaphor, the desire to keep fighting, to be brave, can encourage doctors and patients to sign up to treatments with few or no medical benefits. A culture in which losing or abandoning is not acceptable may lead patients to develop a feeling of guilt. Widening the concept of context, we can understand that in current society – which has a far less military environment than in the 1960s and in which the arms industry faces more public rejection – there is a certain uneasiness with the war metaphor.

On the other hand, society understands the disease differently than it did 70 years ago. Knowledge about it is wider and much more complex. As Nobel prizewinner Harold Varmus said in 2011 on the occasion of the 40th anniversary of the National Cancer Act: 'First of all, I think we've changed the metaphor. It's inaccurate, in my view, to think of a war on cancer as though cancer were a single, individual enemy, nor is the metaphor of war exactly right'.[3] Although in the sample analysed there are only two news items written by doctors, the fact that they used war metaphors indicates their current widespread use among health professionals. Despite the fact that today's comprehension of the disease, as Varmus explains, means that the war metaphor is inexact, it is still a valid way of explaining cancer for health professionals, too.

The view of the patient as a fighter does not seem to be understood negatively because the concept of fight goes further than the military context: It is associated with the ability to keep on going. It can even be comforting. Most people could consider themselves fighters in daily life. Additionally, this fight, understood as an effort to achieve the desirable result, could be considered as a part of the metaphor 'Life is a game', which has a long tradition of use in popular culture (Lakoff & Johnson, 1980; Brooks, 2009). It implies accepting the ordeal with resignation and trying to overcome it, because it is part of the rules of the game.

In the analysed sample, we do not find a substitution of war metaphors with sports metaphors, although they sometimes coexist almost on equal terms. It is also the most used by the patients themselves. If we add to this the fact that the metaphor is not satisfactory for a lot of patients (Wiggins, 2012), maybe we should start to think of a different kind of metaphor to speak about cancer. And, in this sense, the sports metaphor may become a valid alternative, at least in some contexts.

In addition to providing data on the initial research questions, the results of this analysis show other ways in which the media accounts for people with cancer. The heroification of people with cancer, as we have seen, is one of them. As proved by Seale (2002b), newspapers tend to show cancer patients as having special fighting and reinvention skills. In the case of men, Seale claims, those features are courage, altruism, strength, intelligence, honesty and others, and they are present before the disease. In the case of women, however, the disease is understood as a transforming experience that creates a new identity. Nevertheless, in both cases, newspapers tend to attribute imagined superpowers to cancer patients.

Another widely used figure is the personification of the disease. Cancer *strikes*, *stalks*, *persists*, *resists*, *forces*, *reappears*, *hits* and *wins*. Therefore, the disease is not seen as something intrinsic to the functioning of our body but as an enemy equipped with its own personality: ugly, aggressive, insidious, voracious and sly.

Concluding Reflections: New Times, Old Metaphors

If, as Lakoff and Turner (1989) claim, metaphors are such a common tool that we use them unconsciously and automatically, studies like this one can contribute to a more sensible use of them. Cancer is a disease surrounded by many metaphors. As scientific language in regard to cancer becomes more and more specific, to describe an increasingly complex reality, non-expert language looks for new metaphors to explain that reality. However, in the case of cancer, this does not seem to be true.

According to the results of this research, the military metaphor – as was stated by Sontag more than 30 years ago – still prevails. Nevertheless, the sports metaphor is almost as present as the war metaphor, especially in cases such as the ones analysed, in which cancer patients are part of the world of elite sports. There is not, therefore, a single metaphor to understand cancer, and although the military metaphor is still the most common, other ones, probably more appropriate for today's society, are gaining influence. Sports metaphors, and especially football ones, could be useful for those patients who do not feel comfortable with the war metaphor. Although the sports metaphor shares different fields with the war metaphor, like fight (strength) or teamwork (not feeling alone), which can help patients to identify with it, sports metaphors lower the importance of defeat and the pressure to fight until the end implied by military metaphors. Moreover, sports in general – and football in particular – are popular almost everywhere in the world, so the sports metaphor will be comprehensible in many contexts. Finally, everyday language has already included sports expressions and football similes, so their use can help their spread.

The results also prove that in this case study both Abidal and Vilanova were more comfortable with the use of the sports metaphor to refer to their illness. We can observe this, for example, in the letter Vilanova published a day after his resignation. For some, it would be better to focus on learning to live with cancer rather than putting attention on the battle against it. In Campbell's words:

> Why not ask your patients what metaphors work for them? Surely other good metaphors besides sports are out there —art, music, and travel, to name a few. We can start building on these themes, coming up with new messages and ways of thinking and talking about cancer that capture the spirit of the whole experience. We need to convey a more positive, active image for patients living with cancer as well as for their support systems or teams. Maybe the media would even pick it up and change the way the 'C' word is discussed. (Campbell, 2011: 349)

Talking about the media is not irrelevant, because they collect these metaphors and sanction their use. The reflection can, therefore, contribute to the understanding of the social image of cancer and how it can be discussed more adequately.

Be that as it may, our results show that it is still very difficult to reject the use of military metaphors. This image of the war against cancer is so popular that even top sportsmen like Vilanova and Abidal, who avoided using them, were widely discussed in the newspapers using this type of metaphor. In this sense, it would be advisable for the mass media to avoid this metaphorical warfare language and replace it with a description/ explanation that is more sensitive to cancer patients. As has been observed by Hodgkin (1985: 1821), although old war metaphors are hard to dislodge, 'there are many other subjects that might yield additional new metaphors and insights'.

In conclusion, this work confirms that the war metaphor is still deeply rooted in media discourse to talk about cancer patients, even in contexts where other metaphors such as the sports metaphor would be more appropriate. To sum up, this study can contribute to a better understanding of how cancer metaphors are conveyed through the media and how readers receive a specific image of the disease and the people suffering from it.

Notes

(1) Research project 'Lenguaje y cultura de la salud' (CSO2014-61928-EXP).
(2) Periodical audience report by the AIMC (Association for Media Research).
(3) Available in Medscape: http://www.medscape.com/viewarticle/755368 (accessed 24 February 2014).

References

Annas, G. (1995) Reframing the debate on health care reform by replacing our metaphors. *The New England Journal of Medicine* 16, 744–747.

Archer, M. and Cohen, R. (1998) Sidelined on the (judicial) bench sports metaphors in judicial opinions. *American Business Law Journal* 35, 225–289.

Ashton, D. and Feasey, R. (2014) 'This is not how cancer looks': Celebrity diagnosis and death in the tabloid media. *Journalism* 15 (2), 237–251.

Bell, L. and Seale, C. (2011) The reporting of cervical cancer in the mass media: A study of UK newspapers. *European Journal of Cancer Care* 20, 389–394.

Brooks, K. (2009) Life is not a game: Reworking the metaphor in Richard Ford's Fiction. *The Journal of Popular Culture* 42, 841–855.

Butler Nattinger, A., Hoffmann, R.G., Howell-Pelz, A. and Goodwin, J.S. (1998) Effect of Nancy Reagan's mastectomy on choice of surgery for breast cancer by US women. *JAMA* 10, 762–766.

Campbell, M.K. (2011) Cancer is a team sport. *Clinical Journal of Oncology Nursing* 15, 349.

Casarett, D., Pickard, A., Fishman, J.M., Alexander, S.C., Arnold, R.M., Pollak, K.I. and Tulsky, J.A. (2010) Can metaphors and analogies improve communication with seriously ill patients? *Journal of Palliative Medicine* 13, 255–260.

Charteris-Black, J. (2005) *Politicians and Rhetoric. The Persuasive Power of Metaphor.* Basingstoke: Palgrave-Macmillan.

Chiang, W. and Duann, R. (2007) Conceptual metaphors for SARS: 'War' between whom? *Discourse & Society* 18, 579–602.

Clow, B. (2002) Who's afraid of Susan Sontag? Or, the myths and metaphors of cancer reconsidered. *The Society for the Social History of Medicine* 14, 293–312.

Corbett, J.B. and Mori, M. (1999) Medicine, media and celebrities: News coverage of breast cancer, 1960–1995. *Journalism & Mass Communication Quarterly* 76 (2), 229–249.

Cram, P., Fendrick, A., Inadomi, J., Cowen, M.E., Carpenter, D. and Vijan, S. (2003) The impact of a celebrity promotional campaign on the use of colon cancer screening: The Katie Couric effect. *Archives of Internal Medicine* 163 (13), 1601–1605.

Domínguez, M. (2015a) On the origin of metaphors. *Metaphor and Symbol* 30, 240–255.

Domínguez, M. (2015b) Evolution of metaphors: Phylogeny of oil slick cartoons in Spanish press. *Discourse & Society* 26 (2), 184–204.

Domínguez, M. (2015c) The metaphorical species: Evolution, adaptation and speciation of metaphors. *Discourse Studies* 17 (4), 433–448.

Domínguez, M., Pineda, F. and Mateu, A. (2014) Life in a nutshell: Evolution of a migratory metaphor in Spanish cartoons. *Media, Culture & Society* 36, 810–825.

Evans, D., Barwell, J., Eccles, D., Collins, A., Izatt, L., Jacobs, C., Donaldson, A., Brady, A., Cuthbert, A. Harrison, R., Thomas, S., Howell, A., The FHO2 Group, SG Teams, Miedzybrodzka, Z. and Murray, A. (2014). The Angelina Jolie effect: How high celebrity profile can have a major impact on provision of cancer related services. *Breast Cancer Research* 16 (5), 442.

Gibbs, R.W. (2008) *The Cambridge Handbook of Metaphor and Thought*. New York: Cambridge University Press.

Hanne, M. and Hawken, S.J. (2007) Metaphors for illness in contemporary media. *Medical Humanities* 33, 93–99.

Hilton, S. and Hunt, K. (2010) Coverage of Jade Goody's cervical cancer in UK newspapers: A missed opportunity for health promotion? *BMC Public Health* 10, 368.

Hodgkin, P. (1985) Medicine is war: and other medical metaphors. *British Medical Journal* 291, 1820–1821.

Jasen, P. (2009) From the 'silent killer' to the 'whispering disease': Ovarian cancer and the uses of metaphor. *Medical History* 53, 489–490.

Kelaher, M., Cawson, J., Miller, J., Kavanagh, A., Dunt, D. and Studdert, D.M. (2008) Use of breast cancer screening and treatment services by Australian women aged 25–44 years following Kylie Minogue's breast cancer diagnosis. *International Journal of Epidemiology* 37 (6), 1326–1332.

Lakoff, G. (1993) The contemporary theory of metaphor. In A. Ortony (ed.) *Metaphor and Thought* (pp. 202–251). New York: Cambridge University Press.

Lakoff, G. and Johnson, M. (1980) *Metaphors We Live By*. Chicago, IL: The University of Chicago Press.

Lakoff, G. and Turner, M. (1989) *More than Cool Reason. A Field Guide to Poetic Metaphor.* Chicago, IL: The University of Chicago Press.

Lancucki, L., Sasieni, P., Patnick, J., Day, T. and Vessey, M. (2012) The impact of Jade Goody's diagnosis and death on the NHS cervical screening programme. *Journal of Medical Screening* 19 (2), 89–93.

Laranjeira, C. (2013) The role of narrative and metaphor in the cancer life story: A theoretical analysis. *Medicine, Health Care and Philosophy* 16, 469–481.

Marshall, E. (2011) Cancer research and the $90 billion metaphor. *Science* 331, 1540.

Musolff, A. (2008) What can critical metaphor analysis add to the understanding of racist ideology? Recent studies of Hitler's anti-semitic metaphors. *Critical Approaches to Discourse Analysis across Disciplines* 2, 1–10.

Nixon, R, (1971) Remarks on Signing the National Cancer Act of 1971. Online by Peters, G. and Woolley, J.T. The American Presidency Project. See http://www.presidency.ucsb.edu/ws/?pid=3275 (accessed 31 October, 2014).

Palmatier, R. and Ray, H.L. (1989) *Sports Talk: A Dictionary of Sports Metaphors*. New York: Greenwood Press.

Patterson, J.T. (1987) *The Dread Disease: Cancer and Modern American Culture.* Cambridge, MA: Harvard University Press.

Penson, R.T., Schapira, L., Daniels, K.J., Chabner, B.A. and Lynch, T.J. (2004) Cancer as metaphor. *The Oncologist* 9, 708–716.
Periyakoil, V. (2008) Using metaphors in medicine. *Journal of Palliative Medicine* 11, 842–844.
Pragglejaz Group (2007) MIP: A method for identifying metaphorically used words in discourse. *Metaphor and Symbol* 22 (1), 1–39.
Propp, V. (1985) *Morfología del cuento maravilloso* [*Morphology of the Folktale*]. Madrid: Akal.
Reisfield, G.M. and Wilson, G.R. (2004) Use of metaphor in the discourse on cancer. *Journal of Clinical Oncology* 22, 4024–4027.
Seale, C. (2001) Sporting cancer: Struggle language in news reports of people with cancer. *Sociology of Health & Illness* 23, 308–329.
Seale, C. (2002a) *Media and Health*. London: Sage.
Seale, C. (2002b) Cancer heroics: A study of news reports with particular reference to gender. *Sociology* 36 (1), 107–126.
Semino, E. (2008) *Metaphor in Discourse*. Cambridge: Cambridge University Press.
Semino, E. (2011) The adaptation of metaphors across genres. *Review of Cognitive Linguistics* 9, 130–152.
Skott, C. (2002) Expressive metaphors in cancer narratives. *Cancer Nursing* 25, 230–235.
Slobod, D. and Fuks, A. (2012) Military metaphors and friendly fire. *Canadian Medical Association Journal* 184 (1), 144.
Sontag, S. (1978) *Illness as Metaphor*. New York: Farrar, Straus and Giroux.
Van Dijk, T. (2003) *Ideología y discurso* [*Ideology and Discourse*]. Barcelona: Ariel.
Wiggins, N. (2012) Stop using military metaphors for disease. *British Medical Journal* 345, e4706.
Williams, J.T. (2009) Metaphors of cancer in scientific popularization articles in the British press. *Discourse Studies* 11 (4), 465–495.
Wolf, M. (2000) *La investigación de la comunicación de masas* [*Mass Communication Research*]. Barcelona: Paidós.

9 The Discourse of Mindfulness: What Language Reveals about the Mindfulness Experience[1]

Antonio-José Silvestre-López

Rooted in Eastern spiritual traditions, mindfulness practices have lately experienced a great expansion into many areas of Western society, ranging from personal development to education, leadership or clinical practice. The benefits of mindfulness on mental health and general well-being are nowadays reported in an increasing number of scientific publications. In fact, mindfulness meditation is currently a fully accepted procedure in experimental and clinical psychology to treat several health conditions, like stress, anxiety or depression. Although mindfulness has been widely studied in the fields of psychology, psychiatry and neuroscience, its linguistic dimension remains vastly unexplored. This is the niche that the present research sets out to fill.

Mindfulness practices require an open focus on processes of attention and the perception of sensations, emotions and thoughts. The use of metaphor becomes necessary in order to apprehend, mentally represent and 'handle' these phenomena, especially the latter. Cognitive linguistics seems a most appropriate perspective in our endeavour, as its repertoire of tools allows for a detailed analysis of each of these representations in terms of sets of idealised cognitive models (ICMs). In this light, this chapter shows what the analysis of 'mindfulness discourse' can reveal about the mental representations that underlie the mindfulness experience and its practice.

The analysis presented here draws on the linguistic production of the participants in a series of mindfulness courses held at a Spanish university and identifies a series of conceptual metaphors that are recurrently triggered in the linguistic encapsulation of the subjective experience associated with mindfulness practice. These, together with a further series of parameters like image schemas, metonymies and scripts, allow the participants' first-person experience to be modelled and shared with others in conventionalised ways.

In general terms, the results of this analysis provide linguistic evidence of the activation of a consistent set of ICMs whose connected structures in turn cater for discourse coherence and hence the understanding of an often abstract universe of discourse. The study concludes that identifying and learning about the nature of these mental representations can lead to more effective mindfulness teaching procedures, including those of mindfulness-based psychotherapeutic programmes, while also suggesting that analysing this kind of discourse can become a rich source of data for further psychological experiments.

Introduction

Setting the ground

Mindfulness involves being consciously aware of the present moment, deliberately keeping one's attention open to outer and inner phenomena and kindly accepting them without judgement (Kabat-Zinn, 2003; Shapiro *et al.*, 2006). It has also been described as an inherent ability that can be developed by everyone through different kinds of meditative practices (cf. Soler *et al.*, 2014: 1).

Mindfulness is not new; it is, in fact, an ancient practice. Contemplative practices were traditionally relegated to religious cult or spiritual growth spheres, but during the last few years they have entered fully into a wide variety of spheres in Western society including personal development, education, leadership and medicine, to name just a few. Especially over the last decade, the many benefits, effects on brain structure and applications of mindfulness have caught the interest of a noticeably wider range of practitioners and scholars working in the fields of psychology, psychiatry and neuroscience, among others. Nowadays, the benefits and effects of the practice of mindfulness are reported in a long list of rigorous scientific studies (Bishop *et al.*, 2004; Cebolla *et al.*, 2014), and several psychological programmes and therapies – e.g. Mindfulness-Based Stress Reduction Programme (Kabat-Zinn, 1982), dialectical behaviour therapy (Linehan, 1993) or mindfulness-based cognitive therapy (Segal *et al.*, 2002) – use mindfulness as their grounding pillar to treat patients suffering from stress, chronic pain, depression, borderline personality disorder and a range of other health conditions. The number of publications in these fields has now risen to a peak, most of them being devoted to reporting measurable benefits for study participants and positive health outcomes in personal, work and social contexts.

Mindfulness and discourse

As far as the *practice* of mindfulness is concerned, the use of language is perceived in most cases as a hindrance in the development of meditative skills[2] (Hayes & Shenk, 2004: 251); it is an obstacle that must be overcome because its use entails the activation of a range of cognitive associations, biases and cultural filters (Hayes *et al.*, 2001) that may prevent the meditator from properly attending to the present moment and reaching deeper levels of insight.

Moving away from the general conception, a series of studies have analysed the language component with different kinds of aims. Some of them, for example, have analysed the experiences reported by participants in order to learn about the features and qualitative nature of inner phenomena (Hurlburt, 2011; Hurlburt & Heavey, 2006) or as a means to access subjective impressions of the mindfulness experience (Francesconi, 2010). Others have analysed the role of linguistic markers as a measurable component of the mindfulness experience (Collins *et al.*, 2009), whereas some have even evaluated the suitability of the *describing* (verbal labelling) mindfulness facet as related to meditative practice variables (Soler *et al.*, 2014).

Although some may agglutinate a variety of perspectives (e.g. phenomenological, philosophical) to frame their proposals, to date, most of these studies are still primarily confined to the field of *psychology* (Silvestre-López, accepted). It is our contention here that the linguistic dimension of mindfulness remains vastly unexplored and that it can indeed be exploited in many other productive ways, especially when approached and analysed from the field of *linguistics*. This is the niche that the present study, as the onset of a broader research line, intends to fill.

Putting an ineffable experience into words

In the process of mindful observation, meditators become better acquainted with the nature and 'behaviour' of familiar feelings, emotions and thoughts. Among many other fresh discoveries, they also become aware of previously unnoticed urges, emotions or thoughts arising in particular life situations; of their own attitudes towards them (e.g. acceptance, rejection and tolerance); and even of the automatised reactions and unconscious behavioural patterns associated with them. Mindfulness meditation leads meditators through fully direct, first-person experiences concerning not only the perception of outer or inner phenomena but also the particular ways in which they, as 'observers', *perceive* and *relate* with 'the observed'.

While the perceptual experience of outer phenomena can be verbalised with relative accuracy and ease by most speakers (and in most languages), the experientially subjective character of perceived inner phenomena turns out to be harder to describe, as it often reaches *qualia* levels (Chalmers, 1996). Meditators often take pains to put their inner experiences into words, for a wealth of experiential nuances are unavoidably lost in the transition from 'first-person level' (lived experience) to 'third-person level' (communicated experience). Apart from reducing its inherent richness to the limited set of ready-made categories provided by our language,[3] the linguistic encapsulation of this experience automatically brings forth a set of 'cultural moulds' which

– inasmuch as they may not necessarily adhere to the directly experienced in all cases (or rather, to the *conceptual representation* created in the mind of the experiencer) – may also interfere in its felicitous communication.

This inherent difficulty in 'finding the right words' often leads meditators to describe inner experiences in terms of outer phenomena, thereby allowing for concreteness in a rather abstract and intangible realm. It is common, for example, to 'picture' the observer as a passive cinema spectator 'watching' their thoughts, states, emotions and inner events run across the screen, or else to conceive the inner space of perception as the sky and our mental contents as clouds passing by. As a consequence, the use of similes and metaphors becomes a powerful tool in shaping this experience in 'conventionalised' ways that are more familiar to the community being addressed, hence increasing the chances of accurately communicating the experience – or, at least, being roughly understood.

Metaphor plays a crucial role in apprehending, conceptualising (mentally representing) and verbalising the mindfulness experience. However, metaphor is not the only parameter that partakes in modelling the mindfulness experience; a further series of elements team up in order to give rise to both the mental and the linguistic representations involved in it.

Mindfulness and cognitive linguistics

Taking the notion of embodiment as its cornerstone, cognitive linguistics (CL) explores 'the relationship between human language, the mind and socio-physical experience' (Evans *et al.*, 2007: 2). One of its main concerns is the study of the relationship between linguistic and mental structures. The analysis of linguistic data is often envisaged from this perspective as a pathway to access the potential range of conceptualisations that underlie – and are therefore inextricably connected to – language use in several situations and contexts (Lakoff, 1987; Langacker, 2008). In this regard, psychological evidence has shown that, in many cases, linguistic structure not only matches mental representations but also plays a role in shaping them (Boroditsky, 2001; Casasanto, 2013). Thus, some of the most recent CL approaches to critical discourse analysis (cf. Hart, 2015) analyse the ways in which language may be used to create or 'model' particular conceptual representations of experience (for example, those related to social or political events) in specific discourse communities, which in turn give way to a vast array of ideological effects.

In this light, CL seems a most appropriate framework for the study of the features of the discourse of mindfulness and the identification of typical conceptualisations underlying it, as its repertoire of tools allows for a detailed analysis of each of these representations as structured in terms of sets of idealised cognitive models (ICMs) (Lakoff, 1987), including image schemas, frames, scripts and metonymic and – especially – metaphorical models.

Aim of the study

Language may turn out to be a hindrance in the personal progress and practice of mindfulness meditation, but its use is by all means necessary in order to share the experience with others. While this holds true in most contexts, the use of language becomes especially relevant in instructional settings, such as in mindfulness training courses where novel meditators need to learn from scratch 'how meditation works'.

This chapter shows what the analysis of 'mindfulness discourse' can reveal about the mental representations that underlie the mindfulness experience and practice in this particular kind of context. In terms of specifics, drawing on the linguistic production of both instructors and participants in introductory mindfulness courses, the analysis is intended to identify common discursive patterns and typical mental representations (in the shape of different kinds of ICMs) arising in this interactive scenario. The linguistic mechanisms involved are envisaged here as gateways giving access to a range of models that are triggered, shared and even negotiated by the whole (dis)course community in the process of both 'making sense of' the first mindfulness experiences and communicating them to others.

Method

The research presented here focuses on the particular case of the oral interaction of a target group: the participants involved in one foundational (basic level) mindfulness course organised and led by two qualified psychologists at a Spanish university. The course, held in Spanish, was open to the whole university community. Although it had 20 initial enrolments, only 18 participants attended regularly. Out of these, 14 were university students and four were university staff. In this introductory course, the 'novel meditators' had scarce or no experience in meditation (all of them had heard of mindfulness and its benefits, but none of them had practised it before). The total duration of the course was nine hours, in six weekly 1.5-hour sessions.

The oral production of the participants was gathered over the six sessions with the help of a digital audio recorder, which the instructors placed on the floor in the middle of the room. Once the course was over, the recordings were collected and transcribed into a small set of digital documents. The corpus used in this study consists of the whole set of transcriptions.

The contents of the corpus were then analysed manually in a series of steps. As observed earlier, part of mindfulness practice involves placing our attention on the present moment, so that physical phenomena and different kinds of inner events become common objects of perception (Silvestre-López, accepted). The corpus was first reviewed in search of 'common topics' (that is, text areas where speakers talk about common experiences). As a product of this first review, four main general topics were identified (physical phenomena/events, sensations, emotions, thoughts), and the areas of text dealing with them were classified accordingly. The next step involved an in-depth survey of each category, aimed at identifying the linguistic expressions chosen by the course participants to talk about an experience related to the topic. Thus, for example, metaphorical expressions like *'just let your thoughts come and go'* or *'I've got too many thoughts in my mind'*, which hint at the activation of image schemas like PATH, NEARFAR or CONTAINMENT/CONTAINER (Johnson, 1987) and conceptual metaphors like THOUGHTS ARE EXTERNAL OBJECTS (Lakoff, 1993), were identified as involved in the discursive characterisation of the category 'thought'. Finally, a coherent set of ICMs (metaphors, metonymies, image schemas, scripts) was identified as derived from the expressions belonging to each category.

Results and Discussion: Common Representations of the Mindfulness Experience

This chapter presents a small (but illustrative) proportion of the results of this analysis.[4] For the sake of clarity, their description has been segregated into three main sections corresponding to the introduction of a basic scenario where a series of conceptualisations take place ('The basic scenario'), and the characterisation of emotions ('Representation of emotions') and thoughts ('Representation of thoughts') in terms of the interaction of the aforementioned ICMs. Each of the following sections contains a series of 'target texts' (examples for each category) that have been selected in order to illustrate the particular phenomena discussed in them. These are presented in their original language (Spanish). A translation into English can be found in Appendix 1.

The basic scenario

On the space of presence and the observer's model

Attending to the present moment implies keeping an open attitude towards the phenomena that belong to it but also towards the very processes of attention and perception that allow us to 'become aware of their existence',[5] as well as towards the physical and mental consequences that may arise out of their presence in our perceptual space (e.g. urges, reactions, actions, further sensations, feelings, emotions and thoughts).

This perceptual space includes both outer and inner phenomena. It is a space that 'opens' in the mind, body and surroundings of the meditator, extending as far as the meditator's perceptual capacities and field of awareness can reach. The space of presence takes in perceptual information retrieved from exteroceptive, proprioceptive and interoceptive channels and allows for information derived from the 'mind sense'; that is, related to the subjective experience of thinking as a process, of thoughts themselves, conceptually grasped emotions, mental states, etc. Accordingly, the space of presence could be defined as the *experienced space*, where all phenomena of the present moment arise and exist, and where both the physical space (physical, bodily perception) and the mental space (where processes of mental perception and imagery arise) converge into an integrated whole (cf. Silvestre-López, accepted, for a discussion on the nature of this integration).

In this space, both physical and mental 'objects of perception' are integrated as members of the *same* category: phenomena that occur *in* the present moment. This integration is often exploited deliberately in the discourse of instructors, especially in guided meditations. Throughout the course sessions, instructors often guide small meditation exercises intended to bring the participants' attention to all these phenomena by 'reporting' them as they 'happen'. This may be done in a series of ways, but a common one is to create a progression from the most physical and evident phenomena (surroundings, actions, bodily sensations) to the most mental and 'elusive' ones in such a way that the addressees are led into perceiving the latter as clearly as the former. Examples (1–3) illustrate some of these progressions. In (1) and (2), course participants are guided by the instructor in a brief exercise where they need to focus on particular actions and sensations that may arise while moving their body (drawing circles with their wrist in (1) and moving their arms in (2)). In (3), the meditation simply engages them in mindfully tasting a sweet.

(1) Estás ahí, *permitiendo que entre y salga el aire en tu cuerpo mientras te mueves, y permitiendo que entren y salgan pensamientos en tu mente* mientras sigues con los círculos. Y poco a poco vas quedándote en el centro. Inhalas profundo en tu centro, exhalas, relajas los brazos al lado del cuerpo y *permites que igual que entra y sale aire en tu cuerpo, puedan entrar y salir emociones, sensaciones.*

(2) *Y mientras* estamos respirando, sintiendo la gravedad sobre nuestro cuerpo y escuchando los sonidos, *a la vez* vamos a comenzar a mover un poco los brazos y a soltarlos. Sacude manos, hombros … *Y a la vez puedes también ser* consciente de tus pensamientos … utilízalos para estar en el presente, ser consciente de que estás pensando; *no hace falta que* lo pienses, sólo que tomes conciencia. Muy bien, *sacude un poquito más los brazos para soltar los brazos, soltar el cuerpo, soltar tus pensamientos*.

(3) *Del mismo modo que* sentís ese caramelo, cómo se va deshaciendo en la boca, y sentís la sensación en las papilas, la lengua, *del mismo modo que sois capaces de observar esto, cuando surja un pensamiento, observadlo* también, observadlo sin perder la concentración en el caramelo, y abríos a él, abríos a cada pensamiento, a cada sensación.

This sense of progression is reached via parallel structures, as in *'permitiendo que entre y salga aire/pensamientos en tu cuerpo/mente mientras'* (1) and other cohesive devices like coordinating conjunctions and prepositional/adverbial phrases of simultaneity (*'y'*, *'mientras'*, *'a la vez'*, *'del mismo modo que'*) (1–3). Conveniently enough, these also prove to be helpful aids for the instructors in their task of 'collapsing' the novel meditators' attentional limits with as many 'present moment items' as possible (the wider the range of present-moment events upon which the listeners' attention is placed, the easier it seems for them to 'stay *in* it').

It is also common to end these progressions in a sort of climax, where mental phenomena are metaphorically 'fused' with physical ones and hence 'equated' with them at the same level of experience. In this 'perceptual levelling exercise', thoughts are treated as if they were physical objects via the activation of the basic ontological metaphor THOUGHTS ARE OBJECTS (see Navarro, this volume). This case is taken to the extreme in (2) (*'sacude un poquito más los brazos para soltar los brazos, soltar el cuerpo, soltar tus pensamientos'*), where both *language* and *a physical movement of the body* collaborate to enhance the (multimodal) metaphorical effect of granting thoughts physical attributes, as they are (or, at least, are suggested to be) loosened like any other kind of physical tension.

Body motion is replaced in (3) by a different action: observing. Here, the verb 'observe' allows for a subtle progression from a pure act of physical perception to another of mental apprehension: mentally perceiving a thought in the addressee's mind is deliberately equated throughout the discourse of the instructor with feeling (and tasting) a sweet in his/her mouth (in other words, with an object with which the experiencer interacts). Understanding this act of mental apprehension in terms of physical perception, again, is afforded by the presence of the THOUGHTS ARE OBJECTS metaphor in such a way that both thoughts and the sweet can be 'observed'. 'Observing' hence becomes the means through which the experiencer is expected to mindfully access the niceties of both the sweet and his/her thoughts. Yet this use is by no means specific to the domain of mindfulness meditation. It is, in fact, an instantiation of a wider and *culturally extended model* of *perception as observation* grounded on both metonymic and metaphoric projections: our default attentional patterns are usually directed towards the 'outer world', and the main channels through which we gather information are the five senses. One of our five senses, sight, stands out above the rest due to its informational relevance in our everyday 'outer' perception (Sweetser, 1990: 38; cf. also Ibarretxe-Antuñano, 2013) so that, by metonymically highlighting it (SIGHT FOR PERCEPTION), we are licensed to use sight-related expressions to talk about perception and attention in general. This metonymy, however, needs to be combined with further metaphorical processes to yield its full discursive potential – in fact, the metonymic mapping simply sets the ground for metaphorical ones. Thus, the emphasised structure (the subdomain of sight) is made readily available as the source domain for further metaphorical refinements which, with processes of *perception* and *attention* as targets, are shaped in most Western cultures into the *observer's model* (Silvestre-López, accepted). Consequently, this amalgam gives rise to a whole folk model of *contemplative* practices where subjective processes of perception and – by assimilation – attention are discursively structured in terms of the physical field of vision. We could talk in these terms of the ATTENDING IS OBSERVING[6] metaphor as a basic structuring principle for the observer's model exploited in most meditative traditions.[7]

In the light of the previous paragraphs, it seems safe to suggest that metaphor contributes to discourse cohesion in a variety of ways, especially when it combines with more 'formal' parameters like parallel structures and three-part repetitions. Yet it also plays an outstanding role in providing general coherence, as it is the cornerstone for the integration of physical and mental experiences not only in the examples analysed here but also in a wider variety of scenarios.

Thoughts as entities, cultural models and 'mindful models'

The reader may have noticed the different formulation of Lakoff's (1993) THOUGHTS ARE *EXTERNAL* OBJECTS and the metaphor THOUGHTS ARE OBJECTS proposed here. I have deliberately excluded the concept 'external' from the metaphor because it draws a thick line between inner and outer spaces, whereas in the model that is emphasised in this context – that which instructors employ and try to 'instil' in novel meditators – this distinction is blurred in such a way that thoughts are plainly conceived of as *entities* that 'exist' (just like those of a different kind, no matter whether physical or mental) in the all-encompassing space of presence. Thus, while the term 'external' is necessarily implicit in THOUGHTS ARE OBJECTS (for the most basic source for our conceptualisation of thoughts as finite entities with which we interact are the objects surrounding us in the physical world), its exclusion here is intended to mark an additional step taken in the ad hoc modelling of thoughts in mindfulness contexts. In other words, the metaphor departs from the widely accepted cultural model (thoughts as external objects) and takes these external origins for granted, but its new formulation allows the status of *both* thoughts and physical objects as mere 'objects of perception' in the (same) space of presence to be reflected more clearly. As we shall see, in short, the THOUGHTS ARE OBJECTS metaphor is but one of the several ontological realisations of thoughts within the mindfulness model, and it is subsidiary to the THOUGHTS ARE ENTITIES metaphor.

Throughout the mindfulness sessions, and as part of the instruction process, instructors try to generate a qualitative turn in the models with which novel meditators are used to perceiving and conceptualising reality so that some of the 'filters' derived from the 'old' or culturally acquired models are expected to drop and be replaced by more 'mindful' alternatives. One of them is the 'outer/inner world' distinction exploited in most *cultural models*. The existence of this dichotomy in our cultural heritage is most probably rooted, on the one hand, in divergences concerning the ease of perception of external and internal 'events' and the relevance of the former with respect to the latter for immediate survival and, on the other hand, in our cultural/communicative customs when sharing both kinds of experiences. However, while this distinction has an obvious functional load in our everyday action and interaction, its functionality seems to lose relevance in the context of mindfulness instruction and is, in fact, undermined in the 'mindfulness model', especially when novel meditators are in the process of *becoming aware* of the nature and behaviour of their own mental activity and *conceiving* it as one more component of the events or 'contents' of the present moment.

Novel meditators are expected to consciously relate to 'internal events' on a daily basis (that is to say, to attend to their inner world as often as possible), just as they had become accustomed, throughout their whole lives, to paying attention to external 'events' and interacting with external entities. As they learn to do so, simultaneous internal and external activity can be more easily perceived 'in real time' (e.g. the meditator becomes aware of thoughts, emotions or feelings arising or taking place at the very moment of, say, talking to someone or washing the dishes, while also being conscious of the details of the talk or the feel of the water and the dishes while washing them), and internal and external contents begin to be perceived as complementary parts of the same whole.

This new dynamic relationship among the objects of perception leads, in turn, to their categorisation (regardless of their nature) as something necessarily different from the entity perceiving them. Throughout the process of 'mindful observation', meditators progressively gain a deeper understanding of how the 'seer' is different from the 'seen' and how the thinker is different from thoughts themselves; that is to say, they ultimately become aware of the fact that they, as 'perceivers', are different from their percepts and that there is a qualitative difference between the consciousness that is aware of each experience and the experienced as such.

Although this may seem fairly obvious for most physical phenomena, at the level of mental contents this disidentification is rarely fully developed in most subjects. The observer–observed disidentification is, in fact, a desirable achievement in the development of mindfulness skills and is strongly associated with what cognitive behavioural therapies call *cognitive defusion* (Shapiro *et al.*, 2006). The term 'de-fusion' is a very appropriate label indeed, as it intuitively evokes the *fragmentation* of an initially fused whole into at least two different entities, together with the notion of *separation* of one with respect to the other. The metaphor THOUGHTS ARE OBJECTS, as used in the context of mindfulness meditation, also seems a very appropriate one in order to model this disidentification because, by providing thought with an ontological existence, it automatically brings forth the implication that the 'observer' and the 'observed' are different entities. Learning to perceive thoughts as independent entities, moreover, seems a useful way to foster cognitive defusion effects since, after all, modelling thoughts as objects helps the experiencer to 'deal with them' in more familiar ways. For example, adopting the *perspective* of an observer necessarily implies adopting a *vantage point* linked to some kind of *distance* between the observer and the observed; besides helping the thinker to more easily 'grasp' his/her thoughts, this (psychological) distance may also contribute by reducing the influence of potentially harmful thoughts over the individual (Barraca, 2011).

Apart from this basic metaphor, then, the observer–observed disidentification is also modelled in terms of fragmentation and distance, which can in turn be parametrised[8] in terms of whole-part and part-part *metonymic effects* (e.g. mind/mental contents, thinker/thought) associated to the activation of *image-schematic structure* (especially involving PART-WHOLE, PATH and FORCE schemas) (cf. Silvestre-López, accepted, for a detailed account on both parameters). The following sections illustrate how the analysis of language used by both instructors and novel meditators provides linguistic cues on stable conceptual representations of the experience; for example, how 'observers' may take a particular standpoint to deal with 'observed phenomena', and how particular emotions and thoughts may themselves be conceptualised as a different range of objects and volitional entities, each with expectable behavioural patterns that can be parametrised in terms of frames and/or scripts.

Representation of emotions

The representation of emotions throughout the corpus is grounded on a series of ontological metaphors that allow emotions to be conceptualised as three main kinds: animate entities, objects and containers. These, in turn, can be structured in different stages of a script that describes the 'behaviour' of emotions in the space of presence and possible relational pathways (ways of relating) between the experiencer and the experienced.

Ontological metaphor: Personification and objectification

The conceptualisation of emotions as persons (e.g. EMOTIONS ARE OPPONENTS) or possessed objects (Kövecses, 2000) is not new to CL and is, in fact, together with the activation of FORCE schemas (EMOTIONS ARE FORCES), one of the most prolific conceptualisations of 'strong' emotions like anger across languages (Kövecses *et al.*, 2015). Thus, emotions may be described as dominant entities capable of exerting some kind of influence over our internal state. Example (4) illustrates how one of the components[9] of the cognitive model of a *dominant emotion* (that is, the reactivity patterns associated with it) is discursively treated as an entity with these attributes.

(4) ¿Qué implica esto? Pues que probablemente empecemos a sentir una mayor sensación de serenidad en cuanto que las *reacciones emocionales del sistema nervioso ya no nos dominan*, pero al mismo tiempo empezamos a vivir con más intensidad, porque vemos las cosas más abiertamente

In this example, the instructor is describing a stage where, thanks to the process of conscious observation, the experiencer is 'liberated from the dominion' of a stress-related emotion. But throughout the observation process, emotions are most typically referred to as objects that *arise in* or else *come in* and *out* of the experiencer (or his/her field of awareness), as in Examples (5) and (6). These are clear instantiations of the famous CONTAINER metaphor (e.g. THE BODY IS A CONTAINER FOR EMOTIONS) described by Kövecses (1990, 2000).

(5) Permítete el enfado *dentro de ti, obsérvalo,* acepta que eso *está dentro de ti,* no lo rechaces.
(6) Si te *viene* algún pensamiento *ligado* a alguna emoción mientras estás ahí en la postura, permites que esté sucediendo, que esté entrando y saliendo aire, *entrando y saliendo esa emoción*

The objectifying power of ontological metaphors allows us to talk about these entities as objects in physical space, and therefore expressions like *'eso está dentro de ti'*, *'entrando y saliendo esa emoción'* or *'si te viene un pensamiento ligado a alguna emoción'* hint at the activation of a further series of image schemas (not only FORCE and CONTAINER, but also PATH, LINK, PROXIMITY-DISTANCE and CENTRE-PERIPHERY) that may play an important part in the conceptual representation of these experiences.

Our experience with physical phenomena tells us that for an entity to 'fit within' another entity it must necessarily be smaller than the 'container' in which it may fit. It also tells us that smaller objects are easier to control than entities that are 'bigger' than us and that their power or degree of influence over us also tends to be lower when they are 'smaller' than us. This is especially clear when the presence of these entities in our whereabouts may lead to negative consequences for us. Thus, if these entities (potential negative influence) are physically close to us and we are not aware of their presence, they are more likely to end up affecting us in more ways than in situations where we are able to acknowledge their presence and take the appropriate measures.

Likewise, when emotions like, say, annoyance or anger (as in (5)) are at an early stage (e.g. the emotion has just 'appeared', and at this point we may simply notice a feeling of uneasiness or soft irritation) and go unnoticed by us (perhaps because our attention is placed elsewhere), they may grow to have more powerful and intense effects over our physical and mental state as well as our actions. However, if, also at an early stage, we become conscious of these emotions and simply (i.e. without taking any further action) observe them (as objects that are different from us) and their particular 'behaviour' (i.e. the quality of their presence in our field of awareness and their effects on us), their intensity may well decrease up to the point that we perhaps simply perceive them as 'being there', but not directly affecting us. We may therefore be able to perceive them with some kind of perspective or distance, and they might even eventually 'disappear' or 'leave' our sphere of influence.

Ontological metaphor: Emotions as containers

When emotions like those described previously go unnoticed, it is common for the experiencer to 'end up in them'. That is to say, the folk cognitive model for this experience suggests that *'object-like'* emotions may grow to become *states* in which we find ourselves, and that at that point – at least with our ordinary, everyday 'observational tools' – it is often more difficult to 'come out of them'. Both conditions can be represented as in Figures 9.1 and 9.2.

Figure 9.1 outlines a configurational relationship between experiencer and emotion which bears a strong connection with the EMOTIONS ARE OBJECTS[10] metaphor: emotions are conceived of as relatively small objects which can be – or, at least, are perceived to be – 'handled' by the experiencer. This relationship is discursively instantiated in examples like (5) and (6). Figure 9.2, in turn, describes a relationship where the emotion has reached the condition of a state (perhaps over time, or else it has straightforwardly arisen as a state itself). The configuration shown in this figure, therefore, is derived from the EMOTIONAL STATES ARE CONTAINERS metaphor, which in most cases exploits *restrictive* facets of the CONTAINER image schema (cf. Peña, 2003: 267–268). Examples like (7) and (8) instantiate these states.

(7) Cuando estás en la *dinámica de reactividad es difícil detenerla*, pero para la próxima vez posiblemente te costará más iniciarla. Cuando uno ya está *metido en una energía emocional* tanto ya de alegría como de ira, *cuando uno está introducido en ella* […] *detenerla es muy complicado* en ese instante preciso.

(8) Tú te levantas y *tienes* estrés … si tú estás *dejándote llevar* por esa sensación de estrés, emocionalmente, *estás situado dentro del* estrés. Entonces, un primer paso de atención plena es: en este momento, ¿qué es lo que está pasando? Entonces *se abre un pequeño espacio*

en el que te das cuenta, sientes que eres consciente de que en ese momento *tienes* estrés. *Y esto es distinto a estar dentro del estrés: estoy 'un poquito fuera de él'.*

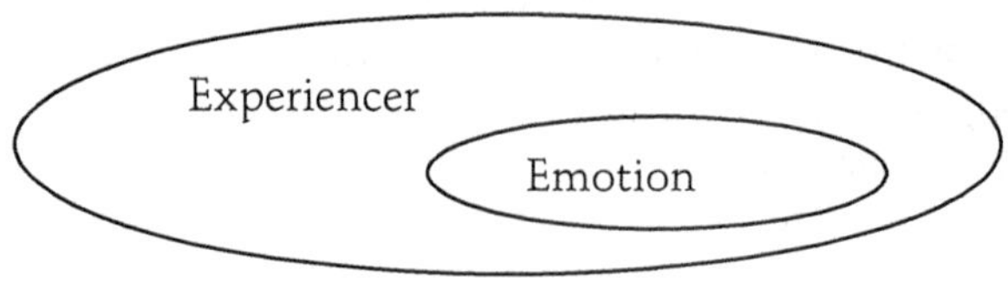

Figure 9.1 Object-like emotion

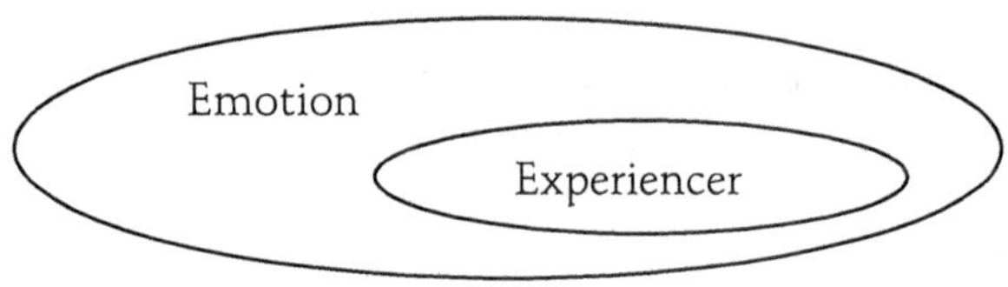

Figure 9.2 Container-like emotion

In (7), the experiencer is described to be *'within* an emotional energy' whose dynamic is very difficult to stop, that is to say, she/he *is* in a state s/he cannot immediately control. This is also the case in (8), where the experiencer is described to be – initially – located within an emotional state of stress. However, becoming aware of this situation may be the first step towards a possible way out. This important step is, in fact, verbalised by the instructor in terms of some of the parameters introduced throughout this chapter (e.g. physical-mental space, distance, observation), together with an explicit distinction between alternative construals like *'tener estrés'* (lit. *'have stress'*) and *'estar dentro del estrés'* (lit. *'to be within the stress'*).

Experiencer and experienced emotions in the space of presence: The script

The range of relationships between experiencer and experienced emotions described so far may be summarised in terms of the following script:

Stage 1: EMOTION AS OBJECT
An object-like emotion appears in the space of presence.

Stage 2a: the experiencer is not aware of the existence of the emotion.
Stage 2b: the experiencer becomes aware of the emotion.

Stage 3: EMOTION AS STATE

The emotion has grown to become a state 'surrounding' the experiencer, or else it appears as a state itself.

Stage 4a: the experiencer is not aware of this state.
Stage 4b: the experiencer becomes aware of the state.

Stage 5: PERSPECTIVE AND CHANGE

The awareness in 4b comes in tandem with the creation of some distance so that the experiencer regains the perspective of an observer and hence the emotion/state slips back into an object-like emotional condition (an entity that can be observed).

Stage 6: INFLUENCE DECREASES

As such, thanks to mindful observation, the power of influence of the emotion may decrease, which may lead to its perception as an object without a direct influence over the perceiver.

Stage 7: EMOTION DISAPPEARS

The (object-like) emotion disappears from the space of presence.

While all emotional states are impermanent, becoming aware of the kind of emotion being experienced and how it is affecting us while it is 'active' *may* (but *does not necessarily*) influence its 'behavioural patterns' or, in other words, how we relate with the emotion itself. Many paths throughout the stages of the script are hence possible, and they do not necessarily follow a linear order. I shall only describe some of these possibilities in the following lines. For instance, the lack of awareness that characterises Stages 2a and 4a may simply allow the emotion/state to take its course (e.g. depending on the emotion, it might become a 'dominant' one as in Examples (4) or (7) or simply develop into Stage 7 with no more consequences). However, becoming aware of the nature of the emotion itself, as in Stages 2b and 4b, may set a different path; in the case of an experienced meditator, for example, Stage 2b may lead directly to Stages 6/7. But it might well be possible for that emotion to 'take over' (even in the case of experienced practitioners) and become a state itself (Stage 3), opening up, in turn, to further possible paths like Stage 4a/4b, where the emotional state persists over time and may still *exert some influence* over the experiencer (i.e. the experiencer becomes directly affected). It may – also over a period of time – evolve as 4a>4b>5>6>7, so that this *influence decreases* as the observation process develops.

Representation of thoughts

While emotions are halfway between the physical and non-physical realms, thoughts are more of a mental reality, and hence our interaction with them is less restricted in certain aspects. For example, thoughts are free from physical limitations (matter is restricted to physical laws, whereas thoughts do not seem to be), and, thanks to our ability for mental imagery operations, they may also be 'handled' in a wider variety of ways. For the same reason, metaphor becomes a vital resource in this respect as well.

Ontological metaphor: Personification

Thoughts may be personified in a variety of ways which allow the perceiver/perceived disidentification to be emphasised not only in terms of perspective and spatial distance between the observer and the observed but also in terms of further human-like interactive nuances. They may be conceptualised as independent entities with free will and manoeuvring abilities ((9) and (10)) and – in the special case of *narratives* (thoughts of a dialectical nature) – as entities that can not only be 'observed' but also 'listened to' (11).

(9) Si algún pensamiento os lleva hacia donde *él quiera*, a su terreno, devolvedlo aquí.

(10) Tenéis que saber que cada vez que *estamos involucrados en un pensamiento, y el pensamiento nos maneja* – ya puede ser de miedo o incluso de alegría, cualquier pensamiento – y en un momento dado hay como un insight que vuelves a la realidad, al presente.

(11) un paso más es, una vez anclados y estando en el presente, *atender* a ese flujo de pensamientos y *escucharlos*, escucharlos no de un modo en que nos identifiquemos con ellos, sino escucharlos del mismo modo que nos sentimos separados de la propia respiración.

Ontological metaphor: Thoughts as objects

In much the same vein, the objectification of thoughts helps us to deal with them as entities that – in combination with other physical and emotional 'objects' – arise and 'move' through the *space of presence* while the experiencer keeps his/her observer's vantage point (12).

(12) Podéis hacer lo que hace la mujer esta, es decir, pensar: '¿porqué yo ahora estaba siendo este pensamiento?' '¿qué sería de mí sin este pensamiento?' *Eso te sitúa en una posición de observador del pensamiento* y entonces la situación a la que te llevaba ese pensamiento, sea la que fuera, fundamentalmente las negativas, el estrés, en ese momento se diluye, *se convierte en una mera cosa que observas, como una procesión*.

The THOUGHTS ARE OBJECTS metaphor allows us to discursively construe negative or unpleasant thoughts as particular kinds of objects (e.g.

figuratively framing them as burdens) and even to provide them with typically physical properties like volume or weight. Accordingly, their degree of influence over us is perceived to decrease as they are 'reduced' or we manage to get rid of their (heavy) load, as in (13).

(13) Tras esto utilizaremos una estrategia de defusión que se supone que es también para *reducir* o *quitarnos de encima* pensamientos desagradables.

As in the case of emotions, thoughts may be metaphorically construed as *object-like* entities that experiencers can manipulate, but also as *containers* in which the experiencers may find themselves. Throughout the following lines, I will use the label 'object-like thought' to refer to the conceptualisation of a thought as a 'small object' with which we can interact (e.g. 'handle' or 'observe' it in our mind's eye, as in (12)), as opposed to 'container-like thoughts', with which I mean to emphasise the conceptualisation of the experiencer as involved in the 'contents' of a thought.

Ontological metaphor: Thoughts as containers

The object-like vs container-like contrast is made explicit in the following example:

(14) Pero cuando tú 'te quedas con un pensamiento' en concreto [...] *ya no estás en el momento presente, estás dentro del pensamiento*. Entonces, es cuando estás pensando ... porque el pensamiento puede ser que tienes que ir al hospital ... y entonces estás en el hospital, preocupada dentro del hospital. Quiero decir, ¿dónde desaparece la sensación de *encerrada* de la mente? Ya no te das cuenta de las otras partes de tu ser, solamente de eso. Eso es 'quedarse con el pensamiento'.
Pero si los pensamientos pasan, tú los dejas, dices: 'permito, no quiero mancharme' ... ese pensamiento pasará y luego vendrá otro y luego otro, y pasarán muchos. Y con el tiempo si tú coges este hábito, pasan menos, con menos frecuencia.

In the first paragraph, an instructor is describing the experience of being 'involved' *in* a container-like thought (*'estás dentro del pensamiento'*) and focuses on the idea that once we are in it, we can access and pay attention to its contents (e.g. being at a hospital), but simultaneously we also 'lose track' of many other details that compose the present moment, that is, of the 'real' situation in which we are actually involved (e.g. having a shower at home).

Apart from the metaphor used in the discourse of the instructor, the reader may have also noticed the activation of the WHOLE-FOR-PART metonymy

EXPERIENCER FOR ATTENTION. Obviously, it is only part of the experiencer, that is, his/her attention or consciousness, and not other parts like their body that can be 'caught by/in a thought'. This is a common, everyday-language metonymy that is often found in the verbalisation of this kind of experience (e.g. *'si algún pensamiento os lleva.'* (9); *'cada vez que estamos involucardos en un pensamiento'* (10)), but in this example it also allows us to understand expressions like *'encerrada en la mente'* or *'ya no te das cuenta de otras partes de tu ser'*. The metonymy also explains why we can still be 'semi-conscious' of the present, physical reality while being 'involved' in a 'thought'.

As in the case of state/container-like emotions, becoming aware of the fact that 'we have been caught by a thought' is just the first step to 'get out of them'. This is the contrast established in the second paragraph of Example (14): object-like thoughts come in tandem with the observer's perspective, and therefore some kind of psychological distance that allows the observer not to 'go with them' (*'marcharme'*) is also implied.

The dynamics of envisaging thoughts as objects in the space of presence and how the experiencer may become involved in their contents are further specified in the script provided in the following section, but at least two main metaphorical projections are necessary for this script to work.

The first one reads THE PRESENT MOMENT, THE PAST AND THE FUTURE ARE CONTAINERS. This metaphor allows us to deal with our experiences of events related to the present moment, the past and the future as *separate* spaces. This yields a wide series of expressions where thoughts carry the experiencer to a *different* (even distant) place (e.g. *'un pensamiento nos lleva [...] a su terreno'* (9); *'la situación a la que te llevaba ese pensamiento'* (12)), even with the additional entailment (licensed from the CONTAINER image schema logic) that when the experiencer is 'in a thought', she/he is not in the present moment (e.g. *'ya no estás en el momento presente, estás dentro del pensamiento'* (14)). The contrast between different spaces/containers is made even more apparent in examples like (15) (*'aquí/fuera de aquí'*), and also throughout the last lines in (16) (*'nos llevaban hacia un lugar en el futuro'*).

(15) Sigo *aquí*, con la atención *aquí*, en este momento. Puede que algún pensamiento me *lleve fuera de aquí*. Me doy cuenta de ello y miro esa sensación.

The second metaphor is, in fact, a further specification of the container metaphor; that is to say, THOUGHTS ARE OBJECTS can be further specified as THOUGHTS ARE CONTAINER-LIKE OBJECTS, and even as a particular kind of container: THOUGHTS ARE CONTAINERS OF THE FUTURE AND THE PAST. Thus, while thoughts are still 'objects' that arise (and exist) in the space of presence (the present moment), as such, they can be conceived of as points of access or 'gateways' towards past or future events/containers. In other words, accessing the interior of an object-like thought means metonymically leaving the present moment to mentally 'access' past or future events.

As we are necessarily physically 'anchored' in the present, we are able to 'leave our thoughts' and bring our attention back to the present moment over and over again. Thus, the present moment is conceived of in this context as the only 'real space', whereas the past and the future are simply mental 'projections', that is, 'smaller spaces' that only exist in our mind and which can only be accessed from the present moment (future and past, therefore, are subsidiary to the present moment). The present moment, therefore, is often equated with 'reality' in a wide series of expressions, as in Examples (10) and (16) (*'vuelves/volved otra vez a la realidad, al presente'*).

(16) Si surgen pensamientos, daos cuenta de cuándo esos pensamientos os han impedido atender a la actividad [que estabais realizando], y volved otra vez a la realidad, al presente. Cada vez que hagamos esto estamos avanzando, tomamos conciencia de cómo el pensamiento nos ha *invadido, nos ha absorbido,* y volvemos otra vez a lo que estamos haciendo. De ese modo aprendemos a elegir, a elegir estar en el presente.
Estamos aquí, en el presente, y poco a poco, si vamos ampliando la frecuencia con la que tenemos esas experiencias cada vez nos será más fácil estar concentrados en lo que hacemos en cada instante, en cada momento, y al mismo tiempo nos será más fácil identificar qué significan para nosotros *cada uno de esos pensamientos que nos estaban absorbiendo y nos llevaban hacia un lugar en el futuro.*

Experiencer and experienced thoughts in the space of presence: The script

Example (16) is a good example in that it very succinctly summarises most of the stages described in the following script:

Stage 1: THOUGHT AS OBJECT
An 'object-like' thought appears in the space of presence.

Stage 2: EXPERIENCER: UNAWARE
The experiencer is not aware of the existence of this thought.

Stage 2a: the thought may not exert a significant influence over the experiencer.
Stage 2b: the thought may exert some sort of influence over the experiencer and may bring with it further thoughts, emotional states and/or particular kinds of behaviours (e.g. shouting at someone).

Stage 3: EXPERIENCER: AWARE
The experiencer is aware of the presence of the thought.

Stage 3a: the thought catches the experiencer's attention, s/he may analyse its nature, but this awareness allows the experiencer to keep a distance (perspective of the observer) so that s/he does not become fully involved in its contents.
Stage 3b: the thought is powerful and influential enough for the experiencer – even while being aware of its presence – to become involved in its contents.

Stage 4: THOUGHT AS CONTAINER
The experiencer is fully involved in the contents of the thought, i.e. the thought is conceptualised as a container whose contents deal with past experiences (e.g. memories of any kind, automatised and/or dialectal judgements about the present experience) or the future (e.g. worries, expectations, future situations).

Stage 5: PERSPECTIVE AND CHANGE
The experiencer acknowledges that s/he is involved in a thought. This realisation allows her/him to regain the observer's perspective (vantage point, distance) and therefore the 'container-like thought' changes into an 'object-like thought' condition (this leads to Stage 3a).

Stage 6: INFLUENCE DECREASES
Through mindful observation, the perception of an object-like thought allows the experiencer to experience it more clearly as an entity that is different from her/himself. The power of influence of the thought over the experiencer decreases (although this may not necessarily happen immediately).

Stage 7: THOUGHT DISAPPEARS
The thought disappears from the space of presence.

Throughout the first paragraph in (16), for example, thoughts are conceived of as entities that arise in the present moment while the experiencer is supposed to be focusing on a particular kind of task (e.g. studying) (Stages 1 and 2). Although they are not necessarily negative entities, thoughts are framed here as 'intruders' that burst into the experiencer's space of presence and carry 'her/him' away from it. They are thus conceptualised as potential distractors from the task at hand; the distraction is, in turn, verbalised as 'absorption' (probably due to the power of attraction of the thought), which finds a correspondence with Stages 3b and 4. By recurrently becoming aware of this process (*'tomamos conciencia [...] y volvemos otra vez a lo que estábamos haciendo'*) (Stage 5), the power of influence of thoughts over the experiencer may decrease (Stage 6) up to the point that many of these thoughts may disappear (Stage 7). This is, in fact, an extremely important process in mindfulness training and, as described throughout the second paragraph, it may progressively allow the novel meditator to more easily become disentangled from thoughts and more conscious of the present moment.

Conclusions

In this chapter, I have unveiled some of the vast array of potential mental representations that underlie the mindfulness experience through the analysis of the linguistic production of the participants in a foundational-level training course. I have provided a basic introduction to the so-called space of presence, how some of the objects of perception are discursively described to interact and how the experiencers are described to relate with some of them (emotions and thoughts). This interaction has been described in terms of a series of parameters that have long been accepted within the CL community: ICMs. Ontological metaphor, metonymy, image schemas and scripts have been shown to combine and provide for discourse coherence and hence understanding among the course participants, which suggests that adopting a CL perspective to the analysis of mindfulness discourse may bring several kinds of benefits to mindfulness research and practice.

The ICMs so far identified are those used discursively in the communication of the mindfulness experience to third persons. As such, they may not directly reflect the exact mental representations derived from first-person experiences. However, inasmuch as language use may influence conceptualisation (Boroditsky, 2001; Casasanto, 2013), the *recurrent* use of a series of discursive devices (e.g. the linguistic exploitation of a particular metaphor as opposed to another) may well have a bearing on the conceptual representations created in the mind of novel meditators. A conscious and deliberate selection of linguistic resources therefore seems a desirable practice on the part of mindfulness teachers and practitioners, as it may lead to better learning outcomes and, hence, more efficient practices and faster progress.

As it is derived from a small case study, the analysis presented here is just a small example of a potentially larger diversity of discourse resources and conceptualisations that can be found in a wider array of mindfulness contexts. However, it is also a first step towards an understanding of the features of the discourse of mindfulness in instructional settings, which may eventually lead – when more representative data samples are analysed – to a systematised classification of conceptualisations and linguistic realisations derived from them.

Two major research lines open up here. The first one envisages this classification as an inventory of items available for further practical and research purposes. That is to say, it may be exploited by practitioners to 'work upon' several dimensions of the experience in more productive ways throughout their mindfulness courses, but it may also be used as a source of data for experimental testing. In this case, particular construals, conceptual configurations and associated linguistic expressions within this inventory may be deliberately selected and exploited in a diversity of settings in order to test their effects (e.g. learning ease, practice efficiency, mindfulness skill development, health improvement, etc.) throughout different mindfulness communities and contexts (from foundational or advanced training courses for a general audience to mindfulness-based programmes aimed at treating particular health conditions).

Along the second line of research, the classification may be envisaged as a 'state-of-the-art' catalogue of recurrent conceptualisations from which – more conveniently based on the results extracted from the first line – a *brand-new* series of deliberate, novel metaphors (or more complex sets of ICMs) can be generated ad hoc in order to attain specific aims. Thus, some of them might focus, for example, on promoting cognitive defusion effects via the activation of particular construals exploiting the metaphorical/psychological distance between the observer and the observed. Others might be concerned with the creation of metaphor systems which help to 'frame' the mindfulness experience according to the needs of particular target mindfulness groups (e.g. groups of different ages, shared knowledge, social background/needs or psychological profile or even groups with specific health conditions).

All in all, further research is needed in the line opened up in this chapter, as the piece of research presented here is but a small contribution from the field of linguistics to the realm of mindfulness.

Notes

(1) Research for this chapter has been carried out and funded under the project P1.1A2014-2.

(2) Although mindfulness is more like a trait or a state we can all develop and experience, it is often associated with meditative practices (mediation is one way of attaining mindfulness). As this chapter deals with mindfulness training, which also involves meditation, 'mindfulness meditation' will be used here in a broad sense to cover mindfulness training aspects, and mindfulness practitioners will also be loosely referred to as 'meditators'.

(3) In this regard, different languages may offer different degrees of difficulty; due to its cultural background, for example, the Pali language offers a wider range of (non-metaphorical) vocabulary than, say, English or Spanish to describe meditation-related experiences.

(4) Due to space restrictions, only two of the aforementioned categories (those which require higher levels of conceptual modelling in terms of ICM interaction) are addressed in this chapter.

(5) These include 'the qualitative way' in which we are attending to, say, sounds in our environment and even whether we are able to mentally perceive potential mental connections, images or thoughts that these stimuli may be triggering at the moment of their perception.

(6) It is important to highlight here the *volitional* component of 'observing' (where the observer is actively involved in the process of observation) as opposed to that

of 'seeing', and its direct relationship with the *active* component of 'attending' (consciously, mindfully paying attention to) as compared to the more 'passive' nature of 'perceiving'.

(7) Cf. Ibarretxe-Antuñano (2013) for a discussion on similar (but slightly different) kinds of metaphor – perceptual metaphors like KNOWING IS SEEING – and their cultural import.

(8) How these parameters combine is a matter of the application of *construal principles* in each case (cf. Langacker, 2008: 55–78, especially dimensions like *focusing* and *perspective*).

(9) Cf. Kövecses (1990: 182–186, 2000: 58–59) for a detailed description of the different components involved in the prototypical ICM of emotions).

(10) The reader may have noticed that the EMOTIONS ARE OBJECTS metaphor allows for entailments like motor interaction and manipulation, which are a crucial component in the mental modelling of emotions in mindfulness contexts, but which are not necessarily emphasised in a potential metaphorical alternative: PEOPLE ARE CONTAINERS FOR EMOTIONS (Kövecses, 2000; Peña, 2003).

References

Barraca, J. (2011) ¿Aceptación o control mental? Terapias de aceptación y *mindfulness* frente a las técnicas cognitivo-conductuales para la eliminación de pensamientos intrusos. *Análisis y Modificación de Conducta* 37, 43–63.

Bishop, S.R., Lau, M., Shapiro, S., Carlson, L., Anderson, N.D., Carmody, J., Segal, Z.V., Abbey, S., Speca, M., Velting, D. and Devins, G. (2004) Mindfulness: A proposed operational definition. *Clinical Psychology: Science and Practice* 11 (3), 230–241.

Boroditsky, L. (2001) Does language shape thought? English and Mandarin speakers' conceptions of time. *Cognitive Psychology* 43 (1), 1–22.

Casasanto, D. (2013) Development of metaphorical thinking: The role of language. In M. Borkent, B. Dancygier and J. Hinnell (eds) *Language and the Creative Mind* (pp. 3–18). Stanford, CA: CSLI Publications.

Cebolla, A., García-Campayo, J. and Demarzo, M. (eds) (2014) *Mindfulness y Ciencia. De la Tradición a la Modernidad*. Madrid: Alianza.

Chalmers, D. (1996) *The Conscious Mind. In Search of a Fundamental Theory*. Oxford: Oxford University Press.

Collins, S., Chawla, N., Hsu, S.H., Grow, J., Otto, J. and Marlatt, G. (2009) Language-based measures of mindfulness: Initial validity and clinical utility. *Psychology of Addictive Behaviors* 23 (4), 743–774.

Evans, V., Bergen, B.K. and Zinken, J. (eds) (2007) *The Cognitive Linguistics Reader (Advances in Cognitive Linguistics)*. London/Oakville, CT: Equinox.

Francesconi, D. (2010) The embodied mind: Mindfulness meditation as experiential learning in adult education. PhD thesis, University of Trento.

Hart, C. (2015) Discourse. In E. Dabrowska and D. Divjak (eds) *Handbook of Cognitive Linguistics* (pp.322–346). Berlin/Boston: Mouton de Gruyter.

Hayes, S., Barnes-Holmes, D. and Roche, B. (eds) (2001) *Relational Frame Theory: A Post-Skinnerian Account of Human Language and Cognition*. New York: Plenum Press.

Hayes, S. and Shenk, C. (2004) Operationalizing mindfulness without unnecessary attachments. *Clinical Psychology: Science and Practice* 11, 249–254.

Hurlburt, R.T. (2011) *Investigating Pristine Inner Experience: Moments of Truth*. Cambridge: Cambridge University Press.

Hurlburt, R.T. and Heavey, C.L. (2006) *Exploring Inner Experience*. New York: John Benjamins.

Ibarretxe-Antuñano, I. (2013) The relationship between conceptual metaphor and culture. *Intercultural Pragmatics* 10 (2), 315–339.
Johnson, M. (1987) *The Body in the Mind*. Chicago, IL: Chicago University Press.
Kabat-Zinn, J. (1982) An outpatient program in behavioral medicine for chronic pain patients based on the practice of mindfulness meditation: Theoretical considerations and preliminary results. *General Hospital Psychiatry* 4, 33–47.
Kabat-Zinn, J. (2003) Mindfulness-based interventions in context: Past, present, and future. *Clinical Psychology: Science and Practice* 10, 144–156.
Kövecses, Z. (1990) *Emotion Concepts*. New York: Springer-Verlag.
Kövecses, Z. (2000) *Metaphor and Emotion*. Cambridge: Cambridge University Press.
Kövecses, Z., Szelíd, V., Nucz, E., Blanco-Carrion, O., Arika, E. and Szabó, R., (2015) Anger metaphors across languages: A cognitive-linguistic perspective. In R. Heredia and A.B. Cieślicka (eds) *Bilingual Figurative Language Processing* (pp. 341–367). Cambridge: Cambridge University Press.
Lakoff, G. (1987) *Women, Fire, and Dangerous Things: What Categories Reveal About the Mind*. Chicago, IL: University of Chicago Press.
Lakoff, G. (1993) The syntax of metaphorical semantic roles. In J. Pustejovsky (ed.) *Semantics and the Lexicon* (pp. 27–36). Dordrecht: Kluwer Academic Publishers.
Langacker, R. (2008) *Cognitive Grammar. A Basic Introduction*. Oxford: Oxford University Press.
Linehan, M. (1993) *Cognitive-Behavioral Treatment of Borderline Personality Disorder*. New York: Guilford Press.
Peña, S. (2003) *Topology and Cognition: What Image-Schemas Reveal about the Metaphorical Language of Emotions*. München: Lincom.
Segal, Z.V., Williams, J.M.G. and Teasdale, J.D. (2002) *Mindfulness-Based Cognitive Therapy for Depression: A New Approach for Preventing Relapse*. New York: Guilford Press.
Shapiro, S.L., Carlson, L.E., Astin, J.A. and Freedman, B. (2006) Mechanisms of mindfulness. *Journal of Clinical Psychology* 62, 373–386.
Silvestre-López, A.J. (accepted) Metáfora y metonimia en la construcción del espacio conceptual y lingüístico en la práctica de la atención plena. *Anuario de Letras*.
Soler, J., Cebolla, A., Feliu-Soler, A., Demarzo, M.M.P., Pascual, J.C., Baños, R. and García-Campayo, J. (2014) Relationship between meditative practice and self-reported mindfulness: The MINDSENS Composite Index. *PLoS ONE* 9 (1), e86622.
Sweetser, E. (1990) *From Etymology to Pragmatics. Metaphorical and Cultural Aspects of Semantic Structure*. Cambridge: Cambridge University Press.

Appendix 1

Translation of examples

(1) There you are, letting air go in and out of your body while you keep moving, letting thoughts come in and out of your mind while you keep drawing circles. You can now stay at your centre, from where you can inhale deeply, exhale, let your arms relax, and – just like the air is coming in and out of your body – also let emotions, sensations come in and out.

(2) And while we're breathing, feeling the effects of gravity on our body and listening to the sounds, at the same time we're going to gently shake our arms and let them loosen up. Shake your hands, shoulders

... and at the same time you can also be aware of your thoughts ... use them to be in the present, to be aware of what you're thinking; you don't need to think, only to become aware of this. Very good, now shake your arms a bit more to loosen them up, to loosen up your body, to loosen up your thoughts.

(3) Just like you can feel this sweet, how it melts in your mouth and how you feel the sensation on your papillae, your tongue; just like you're able to observe this, when a thought arises, observe it without losing your concentration on the sweet, and open yourself up to it, to every thought, to every sensation.

(4) This means that we'll probably start feeling a greater sense of calm because the emotional reactions of our nervous system can no longer dominate us; but at the same time we'll also start living more intensely because we can see things more openly.

(5) Let this annoyance exist within you, observe it, accept that it *is* within you, do not reject it.

(6) If any thought ever comes to you as linked to an emotion while you're in that position, just let this happen, let the air in and out, let that emotion in and out.

(7) Once you're involved in a dynamics of reactivity it is difficult to stop it, but next time you will not get involved so easily. When one is already in an emotional energy, of joy as much as anger, when one is within it [...], it is very difficult to stop it in that very moment.

(8) You wake up and find yourself stressed ... if you let that feeling of stress take over you, then you are emotionally located within the stress. A first mindful step is [to ask]: in this moment, what's going on? Then a small space opens up where you realise, you feel that you are aware that you're stressed in that moment. And this is different from being within the stress: I'm 'slightly out of it'.

(9) If a thought carries you away wherever it wants, to its sphere of influence, bring it back here.

(10) You must know that every time we're involved in a thought and we're under its influence [lit. it *'manipulates'* us], and at a particular moment we experience an insight and come back to reality, to the present.

(11) ... one step further is, once we're anchored in the present, paying attention to that flow of thoughts and listening to them, but not listening to them in a way that we become identified with them, I mean listening to them in the same way that we feel separated from our breath itself.

(12) You may think like this woman: 'Why was I now being this thought?' 'What would be of me without this thought?' That places you in the position of the observer of thought. Hence the situation to which that thought might be taking you – regardless of its nature, but mainly negative, stressful ones – simply vanishes [lit. *gets diluted*] in

that moment, it merely turns into one thing that you can observe, as in a parade.

(13) After this we'll use a defusion strategy that is supposed to help us reduce or get rid of unpleasant thoughts.

(14) But when you 'remain in' a particular thought [...] you're no longer in the present moment, you're within that very thought. Thus, it is when you're thinking ... for example, a particular kind of thought may be that you have to go to the hospital ... and then you find yourself at the hospital, you're worried within the hospital. I mean ... where does the feeling of being enclosed in your mind disappear? You're no longer conscious of other parts of your being, just of that. That is 'remaining in a thought'. But, if thoughts pass by, you can let them go and say: 'I'm letting go of them, I won't go with them' ... a thought will pass and a different one will come, and then another one, and many will just go by. And eventually, if you get into this habit, fewer thoughts will come, they will pass by less frequently.

(15) I'm still here, my attention is here, in this moment. If a thought happens to take me out of here, I'll become aware of this fact and observe [lit. *look at*] that feeling.

(16) If thoughts arise, acknowledge how those thoughts prevented you from paying attention to the task [that you were doing] and then come back again to reality, to the present moment. Whenever we do this we are making progress; we become aware of how a thought invaded us, absorbed us, and we then come back to what we had been doing. We hence learn to choose, to choose to be in the present. We're here, in the present, and little by little, if we increase the frequency with which we have these experiences, we'll find it easier to focus on what we're doing moment after moment. At the same time we will find it easier to learn what each of these thoughts which kept on absorbing and taking us towards a place in the future means for us.

Index